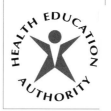

CW00889011

RESEARCHING OLDER PEOPLE'S HEALTH NEEDS AND HEALTH PROMOTION ISSUES

Jay Ginn, Sara Arber, Helen Cooper

ACKNOWLEDGEMENTS

We wish to thank the authors, Jay Ginn, Sara Arber and Helen Cooper from the Department of Sociology, University of Surrey, for having undertaken this review. Thanks are also due to Sarah Harris for her comments and support, and to Chris Owen for his invaluable efforts in the publication of this report.

AUTHORS OF THIS REPORT

Jay Ginn, *Research Fellow, University of Surrey*

Sara Arber, *Professor of Sociology, University of Surrey*

Helen Cooper, *Research Officer, University of Surrey*

HEA RESEARCH PROJECT TEAM

Seta Waller, *Research Manager*

Dominic McVey, *Head of Research*

ISBN 0 7521 1021 7

© Health Education Authority, 1997

First published 1997
Health Education Authority
Hamilton House
Mabledon Place
London WC1H 9TX

Text composition Ken Brooks
Printed in Great Britain

CONTENTS

FOREWORD

The health of older people has sometimes been treated as less important than that of younger people, either because older people are considered less productive or because ill health is deemed an inevitable consequence of later life. Moreover, older people are often mistakenly regarded as a homogeneous group which in turn conceals inequalities in this population. This project aimed to highlight the diversity of older people's health needs and health promotion issues relevant to this age group. The review discusses the influence of the physical, social and infrastructural environment on older people's health and emphasises the importance of recognising the impact on health of the structural and environmental factors outside the individual's control, as well as the need to address these at a societal level. In addition, the review makes recommendations for future research and alternative ways of investigating neglected aspects of older people's health needs and attitudes to health and health promotion.

To improve health, the new HEA strategy continues to recognise the need to create a healthier physical and social environment and to work towards reducing health inequalities in population groups such as older people. It emphasises the need for a national strategy that creates the conditions in which people and communities can take control over their own health. To contribute to this objective, the HEA has in place a three-year strategy to develop the knowledge base of health promotion and to identify innovative approaches. This review, commissioned by the HEA, is part of the wider programme of research which will contribute towards meeting these strategic objectives. The recommendations from this research and the report from the HEA Expert Advisory Group on Older People and Health Promotion will be invaluable in helping to map out the future research agenda for this population.

Dominic McVey
Head of Research
Health Education Authority

EXECUTIVE SUMMARY

Part I   Influences on older people's health

Older people's health has become a matter of increasing interest, fuelled by increasing longevity and a concern that this is matched by increased years of healthy life. The health of older people has sometimes been treated as less important than that of younger people, either because older people are considered unproductive or because ill health is deemed an inevitable concomitant of later life, especially over age 75. Others argue that efforts to improve older people's health are justified.

Older people are targeted in the European Union's health promotion policy and by the World Health Organisation, which aims for 'a sustained and continuing improvement in the health of all people aged 65 years and over'. In the US, older people have become a target group for health promotion (Hickey and Stilwell, 1991), stimulating research and conceptual thinking on health issues in later life (Berg and Kassels, 1990; Kane, Grimley Evans and Macfadyen, 1990).

It is increasingly recognised that the concept of health should include a sense of wellbeing and that this is related to older people's satisfaction with social aspects of their life and the supportive quality of their environment.

Older people are highly diverse in terms of their bodily, psychological, social and material resources; policies to improve health must take account of social structural factors, differentiating according to gender, social class and ethnicity.

Increased life expectancy has been accompanied by higher rates of self-reported chronic illness but it is suggested that reporting rates are raised by factors unrelated to physical health. The question of whether morbidity is becoming expanded or compressed remains uncertain, depending on whether self-reported measures are used or the more objective measure of functional abilities.

In spite of association of advancing age with poorer health, age alone is a poor predictor of health. Morbidity, especially functional disability rates, is related to previous occupational class, to current material circumstances, to gender, ethnicity and area of residence. However, there is no consensus as to whether ethnic deficits in health expectancy stem from cultural practices or from the tendency of ethnic minorities to be materially disadvantaged. Structural disadvantage can be viewed as causing premature ageing in its adverse effects on health. Some of the policy implications of the class gradient in health for younger people – improvements in living standards, housing and the local environment – apply equally to the older population.

In some aspects of behaviour, such as smoking and drinking, older people's lifestyle is healthier than that of people aged under 65, while in terms of diet there is little difference according to age. Not surprisingly, older people's physical activity is less than that of younger people, and is lowest among older women. Among older people, those aged over 75 are less likely to smoke or consume excess alcohol than those aged 65–74 but the older group are more likely than the younger to take insufficient exercise. Diets are more health-oriented among older women than men and older women are less likely than men to exceed recommended alcohol limits. Older men's smoking declined more than women's between 1991 and 1994, almost eliminating the gender difference in the rate of smoking in later life. Class differences in lifestyle are also evident, with older men and women in a non-manual occupational group having a healthier diet. Information on older people's smoking and alcohol consumption according to their social class is not available in the Health Survey for England nor the Health and Lifestyle Surveys.

Longitudinal research shows that older people have modified their behaviour in terms of smoking, alcohol, exercise and type of diet. A decline in psychosocial health is likely to stem from loss of supportive social roles and relationships, as in widowhood. Widows are a particularly vulnerable group, lacking either the social, caring and financial resources of married women or the supportive social networks built up by single women.

While the evidence of lifestyle change among older people indicates that the risk of cardiovascular disease, stroke, certain cancers, cirrhosis and fractures will decline, it is less clear that the incidence and impact of other common and distressing conditions of later life, such as arthritis, impaired hearing or vision and Alzheimer's Disease, can be reduced by behavioural change. Some writers have pointed out the danger that a culture of health promotion centred mainly on individual behavioural change may lead to older people being blamed for their illness (Nettleton, 1996; Sidell, 1995). Many of the causes of ill health are outside the individual's control, including the socioeconomic factors outlined in Chapter 2 and the nature of the local community, as discussed in Chapter 4.

The influence of the local physical, social and infrastructural environment on older people's health has been little researched. In health care, ageist assumptions and practices have been detrimental to older people's health in several ways, ranging from the cuts in continuing care beds in hospitals to lack of knowledge of how age affects the response to prescribed medicines. Scope for action by local authorities to improve older people's health includes reducing local physical hazards to health; ensuring availability and affordability of domiciliary social services, day centres, educational, social and leisure facilities; fostering a positive social environment; and providing health education and promotion programmes designed in consultation with older people.

We conclude that promoting older people's health requires recognition of the impact on health of structural and local environmental factors outside the individual's control; health promotion must therefore be addressed not only at the level of individual behaviour but also at the societal level, with social policies to improve older people's standard of living and access to appropriate health and social care.

Part II   Researching older people's health promotion

There is a range of survey data available for secondary analysis, allowing exploitation of the potential of high quality data on nationally representative samples of the older population, saving costs and time. The largest datasets, namely the General Household Survey (GHS) and the Health Survey for England (HSE) permit a full analysis of the health of the older population that can be related to a wide range of social and economic indicators. Attitudinal information is available in surveys such as the Health Education and Monitoring Survey (HEMS) and the Health and Lifestyle Survey of the UK Population (HALS).

The Health and Education Monitoring Survey should be considered for further secondary analysis, although its potential is limited by the upper age limit of 75. The most comprehensive analyses of older people would be based on the General Household Survey and the Health Survey for England which include all older people but exclude those living in institutions. All the surveys discussed share common elements and can be used to complement each other in a more comprehensive analysis of the health of this older age group.

Qualitative research, including in-depth interviews and focus group discussions are of value in understanding how older people define health, what they see as their health needs and how they perceive issues around health promotion. Interviews with frail and confused older people, in both private households and residential establishments, are important if a comprehensive study of older people's health is to be obtained. Interviews with managers and staff of homes would supplement the views of residents. The insight gained from qualitative interviews would help inform the design of a comprehensive sample survey.

New surveys of older people's health and health-related behaviour, with questionnaires designed to address neglected issues, are suggested. Two alternative nationally representative quantitative surveys are proposed: (1) a survey of 3000 people aged over 50, which would include oversampling of people aged 65 and over, and (2) a sample of 3000 people aged 70 and over. For both surveys, a probability sample is recommended based on selection of a national sample of addresses from the Postcode Address File. A short screening interview would be used to identify addresses containing age eligible respondents. Interviewers would need to be trained to be aware of the special issues associated with interviewing mentally or physically frail older people.

A longitudinal survey of older people's health would provide information which cross-sectional surveys cannot provide, in particular indicating whether there is a compression of morbidity in successive cohorts. The British Household Panel Survey includes older people but currently has a limited range of questions on health, while the most recent wave of the Retirement and Retirement Plans Survey, in 1994, has an upper age limit of 76. The Health and Lifestyle Surveys of 1984/5 and 1991/2 show the potential of a longitudinal study in illuminating changes in health, health knowledge and health behaviour, but numbers are too small for detailed analysis and it is now six years out of date. Extending the Health Survey for England to follow up older people with further surveys would enable older people's health status and health behaviour to be traced over time and would illuminate the relationship between morbidity and mortality.

Part 1

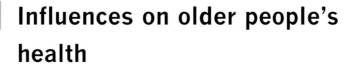

Influences on older people's health

Chapter 1

INTRODUCTION

Older people's health has become a matter of increasing interest, fuelled by increasing longevity and a concern that this should be matched by increased years of healthy life (Sidell, 1995; Bone *et al.*, 1995). In the US, older people have become a target group for health promotion (Hickey and Stilwell, 1991), stimulating research and conceptual thinking on health issues in later life (Berg and Kassels, 1990; Kane, Grimley Evans and Macfadyen, 1990). Older people are targeted in the European Union's health promotion policy (WHO, 1993), while the World Health Organisation's aims for older people include:

- increasing the number of years lived free from disability
- encouraging full and active community life
- prolonging the period of health through better lifestyles in supportive environments. (WHO, 1991)

Good health is a key concern of older people themselves and the main determinant of their life satisfaction. It is essential if they are to continue their many and varied contributions to society and to live independently in their own homes.

The health of older people has sometimes been treated as less important than that of younger people, either because older people are considered unproductive or because ill health is deemed an inevitable concomitant of later life, especially over age 75. Confusion concerning the relationship between age and health, leading to conditions being left untreated, has been reported as affecting doctors more than their patients (Bennett and Ebrahim, 1992).

The objectives of *The Health of the Nation* (Department of Health, 1992) emphasise reducing 'premature death' and specify upper age limits for health targets. This policy implies that improving health is less worthwhile for older people than for younger and is therefore ageist. For example, targets are set for reducing rates of coronary heart disease and stroke among those under 65 and for those aged 65 to 74. Since these conditions are the main cause of death among men and women over 75, exclusion from such targets is discriminatory. Screening programmes also specify maximum age limits, such as 65 for routine breast cancer screening. This strategy has been criticised as lacking a commitment to reducing the burden of illness in the older population (Dalley *et al.*, 1996).

The Medical Research Council is unequivocal in its view that efforts to improve older people's health are justified: 'Older people have the potential to benefit directly from therapeutic and preventive health care strategies, and often stand to benefit proportionately more than their juniors from technological advances' (MRC, 1994: p.62). Similarly, the World Health Organisation's targets recognise the special needs of older people, aiming for 'a sustained and continuing improvement in the health of all people aged 65 years and over' (WHO, 1991: p.33). Yet 'older people' are highly diverse in terms of their bodily, psychological, social and material resources, reflecting the accumulation of experiences over the life course (Arber and Ginn, 1991).

The chief aims of this literature review are to identify the health needs and health promotion issues relevant to older people, differentiating according to gender, social class and ethnicity; and to consider methodological issues in researching the older population, recommending alternative ways to investigate neglected aspects of older people's health needs and attitudes to health promotion. An evaluation of the effectiveness of health promotion interventions among older people is beyond the scope of this review; some of the gaps in knowledge in this area are outlined by Hickey and Stilwell (1991) and a review is provided by Victor (1997). Policy issues are considered by Dalley *et al.* (1996).

A key issue in researching older people's health is the definition of 'older'. This is, of course, arbitrary and the appropriate age range will depend on the purpose of the research (see Chapter 6). To assess the potential for health promotion through preventive measures such as screening and health education, including people in their fifties would bring the impact of retirement and the menopause within the scope of research. For investigating ways of improving coping skills among those with chronic illness, or for assessing the impact of disadvantaged circumstances such as poverty and poor housing, an older age group may be more appropriate. In terms of health decline, the diversity of older people is such that chronological age is only loosely related to 'functional age': working-class people have a functional age some five years older than middle class (Arber and Ginn, 1993).

Definitions and measures of health are related to the underlying model of health – whether this is biomedical or social and psychological. The biomedical model tends to assess people in terms of their anatomy and physiology, leading to a definition of health based on the absence of diagnosed disease. For example, 'health expectancy' – or years of life free from illness or disability – conveniently combines mortality and morbidity into a single quantitative index (Bone *et al.*, 1995). The social model of health is more inclusive, locating individuals in their social context, acknowledging the impact of psychological, social and environmental factors on health and stressing the individual's sense of wellbeing. Thus the WHO definition of health is positive, holistic and qualitative: 'a state of complete physical, mental and social well-being' (WHO, 1985). Health, using this inclusive definition, is hard to operationalise in a single measure but a range of indicators can be used, including clinical assessment of physical and mental functional abilities; number of days of restricted activity; social resources and relationships; economic and environmental resources; self-assessments of health status; and quality of life measures including emotional wellbeing and life satisfaction.

A health promotion strategy for older people will depend on how 'healthy ageing' is conceptualised – whether greater emphasis is placed on longer life expectancy and absence of diagnosed disease, or on optimising functional capacities, wellbeing and autonomy, often within the constraints of established disease. Understanding how people cope with chronic illness is essential to health promotion (Anderson and Bury, 1988; Sidell, 1995) and this issue is most stark in relation to older people with terminal illness, where assurance of access to palliative care or to death with dignity is essential for their sense of autonomy and peace of mind. Health promotion will also depend on the relative importance accorded to social structural factors, individual lifestyle and local community resources in influencing older people's health (as well as on political priorities). In Part I of the review, we consider these three levels of influence on health, defined broadly.

Chapter 2 examines trends in the mortality and morbidity of older people, focusing on differences according to socioeconomic status, gender and ethnicity. We also consider variations in older people's health across regions and local authority areas and how this relates to material deprivation.

Chapter 3 is concerned with how the individual's lifestyle influences health. Research on both physical and social aspects of older individuals' lifestyle which are thought to influence their health is reviewed, drawing on British health surveys and noting changes in health-related behaviour over time. We summarise evidence first on older people's diet, exercise, smoking and alcohol intake, then on social activities, living arrangements, marital and social relationships and attitudes to health promotion.

Less research attention has been paid to how the quality of the local environment may affect the health of older people. In Chapter 4, we identify issues relating to physical aspects of the environment, infrastructural services and social factors in localities and the potential for local authorities and health professionals to promote older people's health and wellbeing.

In Part II of the review, four chapters consider methodological issues in researching older people's health needs and health promotion issues. Chapter 5 examines the potential of secondary analysis of existing national surveys on the health and health-related behaviour of older people. Datasets considered include the English Health Survey from 1991 to 1996, the Health and Lifestyle Surveys of 1984/5 and 1991/2 and the 1994/5 survey by the Department of Health/Ministry of Agriculture, Fisheries and Food of older people, which includes older people living in residential settings (DoH/MAFF, 1997).

Chapter 6 considers the advantages and difficulties of carrying out qualitative research on older people, including in-depth interviews and focus group discussions. Methods of interviewing older people both in private households and in residential establishments are discussed, building on the knowledge of researchers with experience in this area.

Chapter 7 sets out the ways in which new surveys of older people's health and health promotion could best be carried out, in order to address neglected issues. Alternative survey designs are considered for a structured interview survey with older people in private households. The chapter discusses issues of sample size, appropriate sampling frames, response rates, difficulties of interviewing frail or mentally impaired older people and ways of dealing with these.

Chapter 8 discusses the value of a panel or longitudinal survey of older people, in order to trace the process of health change over time and to relate this to changes in health behaviour and in socioeconomic and family circumstances. Problems of using this method for a sample of older people, with a high rate of attrition of the sample through incapacity or death, are considered.

Following the Conclusions, an Appendix outlines the topics covered in existing national health surveys and in relevant sections of other surveys.

In spite of the growth of the older population, British health targets appear to be based on ageist assumptions as to the potential for improving older people's health. Understanding how increased life expectancy is related to older people's functional capacities, independence, perceived health and wellbeing – and how these may be improved – has never been more urgent.

Chapter 2

STRUCTURAL VARIATIONS IN OLDER PEOPLE'S HEALTH

The variation in mortality and morbidity rates according to social factors indicates the scope for intervention to improve health, either through collective or personal action.

In this chapter, we examine some of the research on mortality and morbidity of older people, focusing on differences according to socio-economic status, gender and ethnicity. We also review the limited literature on health variation according to the local environment, including material deprivation and the quality of the social environment.

Trends in mortality and morbidity

Life expectancy at birth has risen between 1961 and 1994 from 68 to 74 for men and from 74 to 79 for women (see Table 2.1). In 1994, men aged 60 could expect to live another 18 years, women another 22. Women's advantage in life expectancy at age 60 increased from 4 years in 1961 to 4.5 years in 1981 but since that time gender convergence is evident, with women's advantage reduced to 4.1 years in 1994. The gender differential in life expectancy at age 80 is smaller, but has consistently increased over time.

Table 2.1. Changes in expectation of life, 1961–1994, men and women, England and Wales

Expectation of life:	1961	1981	1994
At birth			
Men	68.1	71.0	74.2
Women	74.0	77.0	79.4
Sex differential	5.9 years	6.0 years	5.2 years
At age 60			
Men	15.1	16.4	18.3
Women	19.1	20.9	22.4
Sex differential	4.0 years	4.5 years	4.1 years
At age 80			
Men	5.2	5.8	6.6
Women	6.4	7.5	8.5
Sex differential	1.2 years	1.7 years	1.9 years

Source: OPCS (1996), table 12

In line with increased life expectancy, the proportion of the population aged over 65 grew from 13 per cent in 1971 to 16 per cent in 1981, and remained stable at this level until 1995 (see Table 2.2a). It is projected to fall to 15 per cent by 2001, and rise to 17 per cent by 2011 (OPCS, 1996). The proportion of people aged over 85 doubled from 0.9 per cent of the population in 1971 to 1.8 per cent in 1995 (see Table 2.2a) (OPCS, 1996).

Later life becomes increasingly feminised with advancing age. In 1995, the ratio of women to men was 1.46 among all those aged over 65 but women outnumbered men by two to one among the over-75s and by nearly three to one among the over-85s (see Table 2.2a). Because of women's greater average longevity and the tendency for wives to be younger than their husbands (by two years on average), older women are much more likely than men to be widowed. Thus half of older women are widowed, compared with only 17 per cent of older men (see Table 2.2b). This leads to gender differences in living arrangements, with older women more likely than men to live alone and to lack access to informal care in their own home (Arber and Ginn, 1990; 1991).

Table 2.2. Demographic characteristics of women and men aged 65 and over, England and Wales

	All	Women	Men	Sex ratio (Women/Men)
(a) % of population				
1971				
% over 65	13.4%	16.1%	10.6%	1.61
% over 75	4.8%	6.4%	3.1%	2.15
% over 85	0.9%	1.3%	0.5%	2.90
1995				
% over 65	15.9%	18.5%	13.2%	1.46
% over 75	7.1%	9.1%	5.0%	1.89
% over 85	1.8%	2.7%	0.9%	2.95
(b) Marital status	%	%	%	
1992				
Married	52.1	38.4	72.3	0.79
Widowed	36.2	49.2	16.8	4.36
Never married	8.1	8.6	7.5	1.70
Divorced/Separated	3.6	3.8	3.4	1.63
	100	100	100	
N (millions)	8.16	4.88	3.28	

Source: OPCS (1996), tables 6 and 7.

For morbidity, rates and trends are more difficult to establish than for mortality. Morbidity rates depend on the measure used, whether self-reports of general health, long-standing illness, limiting long-standing illness, acute illness restricting activity, inability to perform different sets of activities of daily living or use of health services. Sidell (1995) points out the uncertain meaning of health, as shown by older people commonly rating their health as good in spite of having some impairment.

Because the likelihood of both acute and chronic ill health among older people increases with age (Martin, Meltzer and Elliot, 1988; Arber and Ginn, 1991; Victor, 1991), the growth in the older population has given rise to fears of escalating demand for health services. A key question for research has been the relationship between mortality and morbidity. Some gerontologists have predicted that healthier living conditions through the life course will lead to individuals enjoying on average both longer life and a shorter duration of ill health before death – a compression of morbidity (Fries, 1980; 1989). Others argue that acute fatal diseases will be replaced by non-fatal degenerative diseases – a substitution of morbidity for mortality (van de Water, 1997) – so that the duration of morbidity is expanded (Gruenberg, 1977; Kramer, 1980). Some suggest there may be a mixture of both expansion of and compression of morbidity; the process may differ for population sub-groups (Victor, 1991). Which of these scenarios emerges will clearly have important implications both for the welfare of older people and for the future costs of health care and social care. Before examining the question of duration of morbidity, we outline trends in morbidity as measured by self-reported chronic illness in cross-sectional surveys.

Increased rates of limiting long-standing illness have been reported by the adult population, from 14 per cent in 1974 to 19 per cent in 1995 (ONS, 1997a: p.123), although rates show stability since the mid-1980s (ONS, 1997b: fig. 7a). It is striking that the increase over time was greatest for those aged 45 to 64, from 21 per cent to 27 per cent, while those aged over 65 showed a much smaller increase, from 35 per cent to 37 per cent (ONS, 1997a: p. 123). Redundancy and high unemployment among those under state pension age and the financial advantage of Invalidity (now Incapacity) Benefit over Income Support may partly explain the increased chronic illness reported in mid-life. Another explanation may relate to rising expectations and awareness of health over time, later cohorts being more likely to report illness than earlier (Bone et al., 1995). These possibilities draw attention to the socially constructed component in some health measures, which depend on the social context as well as on a person's physical condition.

Acute illness, as measured by reported restriction of normal activities in the previous two weeks, also shows an increase since the 1970s, for both women and men, but is only weakly related to age (ONS, 1997b: table 7.1c). In contrast, acute illness measured by the average number of restricted days per year showed an accelerating increase with age, from 20 days among those aged 16 to 44, to 37 days (age 45 to 64), 48 days (age 65 to 74) and 71 days among those aged over 75 (ONS, 1997b: table 7.14). However, these figures are estimates derived from the reported number of days restricted by illness in the previous two weeks and multiplied by 52 to represent the last year.

Victor (1991) found that between 1980 and 1985 there had been little change in older people's self-assessed general health, within five-year age groups, nor in the prevalence of acute illness. The prevalence of self-reported chronic illness had declined slightly for those aged 70–79.

Using a measure of functional disability, research in the US has found a decline in the age-sex standardised rate of disabling conditions (Manton, Stallard and Corder, 1995): the probability of a person aged 85 or older remaining free of disabilities increased by nearly 30 per cent between 1982 and 1989 and findings from a 1994 follow-up suggest further falls in disability (Manton, Stallard and Corder, 1995).

Due to lack of suitable British data, the Medical Research Council concluded 'It is a matter of profound concern that it is currently not possible to determine whether the health status of the older population has improved, deteriorated or remained the same during the past decades of mortality decline' (MRC, 1994: p26).

Since then, Bone et al. (1995) have published a comprehensive review of the expectancy of healthy life. Life expectancy and measures of health are combined into a single index – health expectancy – measuring the length of life which can be expected free from chronic illness or disability at given ages. Bone et al. (1995) examine a range of approaches to assessing whether there has been a compression (reduction) of morbidity. They come to opposing conclusions, depending on which measures of morbidity are used: using severe disability measures based on activities of daily living shows a compression of morbidity, but using self-reported limiting long-standing illness trends from the General Household Survey from 1976 to 1991, they argue that there has been an expansion of morbidity. Their estimates for the UK have been hampered by the lack of national longitudinal data on health and disability among the older population. Bone et al. (1995) point out that trends in health expectancy will be influenced not only by cohort differences in disease vulnerability but also by increasing recovery from illness states as treatment options expand.

The association of both morbidity and mortality with age can distract from the diversity in health experience within any particular age group. Older people's health is influenced by their life course, in terms of their parental background and behavioural lifestyle, gender, occupation and employment history, housing, marital and parental history, magnifying the diversity associated with genetic factors. Although the probability of ill health rises with age, there is no specific age at which it increases in a stepped or discontinuous way. Thus differences in health within age groups may be more important than differences between age groups. Some researchers have suggested that whether the duration of morbidity is expanding or contracting in later life may depend on gender (Verbrugge, 1984a; Sidell, 1991; Victor, 1991) and class (Victor, 1991).

Class differences in health in later life

Research has established how the distribution of mortality and level of health in modern populations of working age varies with social class (DHSS, 1980; Townsend, Davidson and Whitehead, 1988; Breeze, Trevor and Wilmot, 1991; Jacobson, Smith and Whitehead, 1991; Blane, Davey Smith and Bartley, 1990; Fox, 1989; Illsley and Svensson, 1990; ONS, 1997b) and with gender (Arber, 1987; 1997). Class-related differences in rates of mortality, limiting long-term illness, disability and GP consultation for serious illness apply irrespective of the indicator used – occupational class, housing tenure or car ownership (OPCS, 1986; Goldblatt, 1990; King's Fund Institute, 1994; McCormick and Rosenbaum, 1990; Arber and Ginn, 1993).

Older people have often been excluded in studies of health inequality, as if structural influences ceased to operate after state pension age. However, a few studies of variation in older people's health are available, including age cohort comparisons (Svanborg, 1988) and cross-national comparisons (WHO, 1983), and research has confirmed that the influence of occupational class on chronic illness persists into later life (Taylor, 1988; Victor and Evandrou, 1987; Victor, 1991; Arber and Ginn, 1991; 1993). Arber and Ginn's (1991) analysis of General Household Survey data found clear class gradients within each five-year age group over 65 for both self-assessed health and functional disability, assigning class on the basis of the individual's last or main occupation. For example, within each age group at least 20 per cent more higher middle-class men (managers and professionals) assessed their health as 'good' compared with unskilled men, while unskilled men were twice as likely as higher middle-class men to have moderate or severe disability. The class gradients were also apparent for older women based on their own last occupation (Arber and Ginn, 1991). More recent analysis of the General Household Survey shows that educational qualifications have a major independent effect on older people's self-assessed health. Among men aged 60 to 69 in 1991–2, those with no educational qualifications had twice the odds ratio of reporting poor health compared with men with a degree, after taking account of age, marital status, occupational class and employment status; for women aged 60 to 69, the effect was even greater (Arber, 1996).

In addition to occupational class, current material circumstances have an independent influence on self-assessed health of older people (Arber and Ginn, 1991; 1993). Reporting 'good' health was more likely for those with a high current income, those owning their home or having a car in the household, after controlling for occupational class. For example, older women with a high income were 40 per cent more likely to rate their health as good, compared with low-income women, after controlling for age and class. Disability, on the other hand, was unaffected by current income after controlling for class, although women living in rented accommodation were more likely than owner occupiers to have a moderate level of disability. Arber and Ginn (1993) concluded that previous occupational class is a more important determinant of health among older men and women than current material resources, but that the latter contributes significantly to a sense of well-being. Having adequate material resources is likely to facilitate health-promoting activities, an issue we return to in Chapter 3.

More recent data confirm the class gradient in health among older people (ONS, 1997b). In 1995, 50 per cent of professional men over 65 reported a long-standing illness, compared with 56 per cent of unskilled manual men (class being assigned according to the previous occupation of the head of household). Both men and women living in non-manual households were less likely to report a long-standing illness than those in manual households, a difference of five percentage points (ONS, 1997b: table 7.2). Somewhat greater class differences were evident in the rates of limiting long-standing illness; for non-manual men and women the rates were 34 per cent and 39 per cent respectively, compared with 42 per cent and 48 per cent among manual men and women. Although occupational class had little effect on acute sickness (as indicated by the percentage reporting restricted activity in the previous two weeks), the average number of days per year on which activity was restricted was higher for manual workers (ONS, 1997b: table 7.4). The non-manual: manual divide was apparent among older people for each of the main conditions underlying chronic sickness –

impairment of the musculo-skeletal, circulatory, respiratory, digestive and nervous systems being more likely for the manual group. Only for the endocrine and metabolic system were problems more common among the non-manual group (ONS, 1997b: table 7.13).

Occupational class extends its influence on health beyond the working life, both directly and through its effect on the standard of living in later life. The effect of gender is more complex than that of class; whereas class affects morbidity and mortality in the same way, this is not so for gender.

Gender differences in health in later life

Differences between men's and women's health and mortality are likely to depend on their biological sex as well as on socially created gender roles; since these two sources of health variation are conflated in health statistics and research, we use the term gender to refer to both sex and gender.

Studies of mortality in later life have often been restricted to men (for example, Goldblatt, 1990; Fox, Goldblatt and Jones, 1983) in spite of the preponderance of women among older people. Women's life expectancy at birth is longer than men's in most modern societies, five years in Britain (Table 2.1) and seven in the US (Arber and Ginn, 1991). The gender difference in mortality rates is most marked among the younger elderly, tending to converge with age (see Table 2.3). For example, in England and Wales in 1995, men's death rate per thousand was 69 per cent higher than women's among those aged 65 to 74, 57 per cent higher at ages 75 to 84 and only 28 per cent higher for those aged over 85. Over the past 25 years, the gender difference in mortality rates has declined among the younger old but increased slightly among those who are older. For example, for those aged 65–74, the gender differential fell from 1.93 in 1971 to 1.69 in 1995, whereas for those aged 75–84 the differential rose slightly from 1.54 to 1.57 over the same period (Table 2.3).

The reasons for women's greater longevity are uncertain: Waldron (1976) suggests that 75 per cent of the gender difference in mortality is attributable to behavioural factors, although other writers' estimates vary.

Women in later life show a higher prevalence of ill health on several measures, in spite of their lower mortality, in both Britain and the US (Martin, Meltzer and Elliot, 1988; Arber and Ginn, 1991; 1993; Verbrugge, 1984b). For example, among those over 75, twice as many British women as men were housebound, 22 per cent compared with

Table 2.3. Age-specific mortality rates (per thousand) 1971–1995, men and women, age 55 and over, England and Wales

	55–64	65–74	75–84	85+
1971				
Men	20.1	50.5	113.0	231.8
Women	10.0	26.1	73.6	185.7
Sex differential	2.01	1.93	1.54	1.25
1995				
Men	12.2	35.9	88.8	197.3
Women	7.3	21.3	56.6	151.8
Sex differential	1.70	1.69	1.57	1.28
% Decrease, 1971–95				
Men	39.3%	29.0%	21.4%	16.2%
Women	27.0%	17.4%	23.1%	18.3%

Source: OPCS (1996), table 13

11 per cent, and only a quarter of women were medically assessed as fit compared with 36 per cent of men (Hall and Channing, 1990). Cognitive impairment among those over age 80 is also more likely among women than men (Jagger, Clarke and Cook, 1989).

Research on older people using the 1985 General Household Survey data showed that older women were about twice as likely as men to report impaired mobility, the gender difference increasing with age (Arber and Ginn, 1991). These gender differences in functional disabilities were confirmed by the 1994 General Household Survey (Bennett *et al.*, 1996). Mobility restrictions were low for those aged 65 to 74 but increased markedly over age 85. Among those over 85, nearly half of women were unable to go out and walk down the road compared with less than a fifth of men; 29 per cent of women but less than 10 per cent of men could not manage stairs. Older women were also more likely than men to be unable to perform essential personal self-care tasks. Among those aged over 65, 10 per cent of women and 6 per cent of men could not bath, shower or wash all over without assistance but this restriction applied to nearly a quarter of women over 85. Thus although most older people can live independently, older women are more likely than men to have disabilities requiring help from others, either from health and welfare services or from informal carers.

Gender differences in self-assessed health among older people were relatively modest and were less important than differences associated with class and financial resources. Nevertheless, about 5 per cent more men than women rated their health as good (Arber and Ginn, 1991).

Among those over 75, rates of reported long-standing illness and limiting long-standing illness have been consistently higher for women than men over the last two decades (ONS, 1997b: table 7.1a and b), but among the younger elderly, aged 65 to 74, gender differences have been lower or reversed. Acute illness, as measured by restricted activity in the past two weeks, has been consistently higher for women than men among all aged over 65 (ONS, 1997b: table 7.1c).

The seeming paradox that women have lower mortality but higher morbidity has stimulated academic debate (Nathanson, 1975; 1977; Verbrugge, 1989; Waldron, 1976). One suggestion is that women's higher morbidity reflects a greater propensity to perceive their health as poor. Although this may partly explain women's poorer self-assessed health, the substantial gender difference in functional ability is unlikely to be an artefact. Manton (1988) has shown that older women's higher prevalence of disability is not due to higher incidence of disabling conditions but to lower mortality from them. Older women are more likely than men to have non-lethal disabilities, especially those associated with musculo-skeletal disorders (Verbrugge, 1989), whereas cardiovascular conditions (including heart problems and stroke) are more common in older men than women. For example, in 1994 among those aged 65 to 74, 10 per cent of men but 6 per cent of women reported angina and over age 75 the proportions were 13 per cent and 9 per cent (Colhoun and Prescott-Clarke, 1996).

Women's morbidity disadvantage is evident within each occupational class grouping and age group (Arber and Ginn, 1993). Thus gender has a separate effect from that of class. The relationship of ethnicity to mortality and morbidity rates, to which we turn next, is affected by the tendency for some ethnic minorities to cluster in the lower occupational classes.

Ethnicity and health in later life

Both biological differences (race) and cultural factors (ethnicity) are likely to contribute to health differences between people from ethnic minorities and the majority population. We use 'ethnicity' here to include differences from both these sources.

Research on the relationship between ethnicity and health in later life is less developed in Britain than in the US, where black Americans have a shorter life expectancy than the average for the population (Markides, 1989). However, US blacks aged over 75 have lower mortality than whites due to selective survival – the 'racial crossover'.

In Britain, 'research interest in the health of minority ethnic elders is in its infancy' (Smaje, 1995: p.132), partly because the number of minority ethnic men and women aged over 65 is currently too small for reliable analysis of specific ethnic groups: only 1 per cent of the British population over state pension age were from ethnic minorities in the 1980s (Arber and Ginn, 1991), although the proportion will rise as the ethnic populations age.

There is some evidence of mortality differences in Britain according to country of origin, but the effect varies with age. Among those aged 20 to 69 in the early 1980s, mortality was raised relative to the general population for those born in Ireland, the Indian subcontinent and the Caribbean and African Commonwealth countries, only Caribbean Commonwealth men having lower mortality. However, among those aged over 70, the picture is reversed: all groups except Indian women and Irish-born men and women had lower mortality rates than the general population (Balarajan and Bulusi, 1990).

Analysis of the 1991 Census shows raised prevalence of limiting long-standing illness, relative to the white population, for adult men and women in all ethnic groups identified, with the exception of Chinese (Bone et al., 1995: table 7.5). For London wards, these authors have estimated health expectancy (HE) relative to whites as four years less for black men. Among those from the Indian sub-continent, HE was estimated to be 2.5 years less for men and five years less for women (Bone et al., 1995: table 7.8). They suggest that the lower average HE of ethnic minorities stems largely from the difference in social class composition compared with the white population.

Small-scale research on morbidity among ethnic minority older people is outlined by Smaje (1995). Ebrahim et al. (1991) found that Gujeratis aged over 54 in North London had higher prevalence of chronic illness than a matched sample of whites; Donaldson (1986) found high levels of functional disability among South Asians aged over 65 in Leicester; Fenton (1985) found older people of Caribbean origin had problems with hypertension and diabetes. Blakemore and Boneham (1993) also review research on the health of ethnic minority elders, concluding that their health is poorer than would be expected on the basis of their age distribution.

Research on ethnic minority older people in Britain has raised the issue of their disadvantage in material circumstances (Barker, 1984; Norman, 1985; Blakemore, 1989; Cameron et al., 1989). Because of the association of health with socioeconomic factors and ethnic differences in class distribution, it is difficult to quantify the independent

effect of ethnicity on health. Marmot, Adelstein and Bulusi (1984) cal-
culated mortality ratios according to social class, for adult men from a
number of migrant groups. They found that the expected class gradient was only present for Irish men. Since, for most minority ethnic
groups, differences from whites in mortality did not disappear when
class was controlled, they concluded that 'differences in social class distribution are not the explanation of the overall different mortality of
immigrants' (Marmot, Adelstein and Bulusi, 1984: p.21). However, due
to the small numbers of deaths in some cases, the claim must be treated with caution.

A somewhat different conclusion is reached by Mays (1994).
Observing the persistent health disadvantage of the Irish population in
Britain, he suggests that ethnic differences in health are not primarily
cultural in origin but due to 'selective migration, discrimination and a
disadvantageous position in the labour market' (p.67); for this reason,
he argues that health deficits seen in the black population will also persist. As Smaje (1995) comments, further research is needed to
disentangle the multiple explanatory factors involved in the health of
ethnic minorities, an observation which applies equally to the health of
older people from ethnic minorities.

Among older people, the structural variations in health due to class,
gender and ethnicity which we have outlined partly reflect the effect of
health selection, particularly selective survival. In population sub-
groups with a higher than average adult mortality rate, the survivors
are likely to be unrepresentative of their birth cohort, being fitter than
those who have died would have been. Because of selective survival,
class, ethnic and gender differences can be expected to be less among
older than younger people, narrowing with advancing age.

Locality and health

Part of the explanation for the association between lower social class
and poorer health may lie in the area of residence and factors in the
local social and physical environment. We next examine the relationship between area of residence and health.

Health differences associated with regions have long been established (Tudor Hart, 1971) and recent evidence of the national divide in
health is provided by the 1991 Census (Bone et al., 1995: pp.34–41). In
terms of both age-standardised chronic illness rates and life expectancy, the north and west of England and Wales are differentiated from
the South and East, where people not only live longer but are healthier. A man in south-east England can expect to live 89 per cent of his

life in good health, compared with 82 per cent for a man in Wales. Comparison of health expectancy for different age groups show that the regional patterns persist into later life (Bone *et al.*, 1995).

The analysis by Bone *et al.* (1995) of the relationship between life expectancy at birth and expected years of ill health for each of the 115 local authority areas shows substantial deviation in some areas from the morbidity rate predicted by the overall relationship between morbidity and life expectancy. For example, areas where mining was a major industry, such as Barnsley and Glamorgan, had higher morbidity than expected; raised morbidity was evident for women as well as men, indicating that the local environment rather than the predominant occupation was responsible.

The 'quality' of localities has been summarised in terms of indexes of deprivation, based on housing tenure, overcrowding rate, average household income, proportion of lone parent families, unemployment rate, social class composition of the area and so on (Townsend, Phillimore and Beattie, 1988). We would expect the health of those with long residence in a relatively deprived locality to have poorer health than average. The association of local deprivation and poor health is shown by the raised rates of hospital admissions and of mortality in London's most deprived wards (London Research Centre, 1997).

Summary

Increased life expectancy has been accompanied by higher rates of self-reported chronic illness but it is suggested that reporting rates are raised by factors unrelated to physical health. The question of whether morbidity in later life is becoming expanded or compressed remains uncertain, depending on whether self-reported measures are used or the more objective measure of functional abilities.

In spite of association of advancing age with poorer health, age alone is a poor predictor of health. Morbidity, especially functional disability rates, is related to previous occupational class, to current material circumstances, to gender, ethnicity and area of residence. However, there is no consensus as to whether lower health expectancy among people from ethnic minorities stems from cultural practices or from the tendency of ethnic minorities to be materially disadvantaged. Structural disadvantage can be viewed as causing premature ageing in its adverse effects on health. Some of the policy implications of the class gradient in health for younger people – improvements in living standards, housing and the local environment – apply equally to the older population.

Evidence for the influence of structural factors on health in later life has been outlined but the relative importance of the materialist and the cultural/behavioural explanations of health differences is controversial (Whitehead, 1987). Although class, gender and ethnicity influence the material and social context, favourable or otherwise, in which an individual lives, health outcomes are not wholly determined by structural constraints; healthy behaviour, which is considered in the next chapter, also contributes to successful ageing and the preservation of functional ability.

Chapter 3

PERSONAL LIFESTYLE AND HEALTH BEHAVIOUR AMONG OLDER PEOPLE

In this chapter we consider how individual behaviour is related to health. The value of health promotion for older people has sometimes been questioned on the grounds that later life is inevitably accompanied by ill health, that it is too late to stem degenerative processes arising in earlier life, or that older people cannot change established habits. On the other hand, there is growing evidence that modifying risk factors in later life can still improve health (Hickey and Stilwell, 1991; Edwards and Larson, 1992), that there is scope for improving clinical detection (Davies, 1990), medical intervention (Medical Research Council, 1994), and rehabilitation (Royal College of Physicians, 1992), that older people can be receptive to advice (Karp, 1988; Emery, Hauck and Blumenthal, 1992), and that older people are increasingly likely to report health-promoting behaviours (Swain, 1993a).

In this chapter we review research on both physical and social aspects of older individuals' lifestyle which are thought to influence their health. We thus include research informed by both the biomedical and the social models of health. Although the focus here is on the effects of lifestyle on health, the relationship between behaviour and health is reciprocal in that a person's state of health may influence their capacity for health-promoting behaviours. We first examine survey evidence on older people's diet, exercise, smoking and alcohol intake, including changes over time. We then review research on how health is related to social activities, living arrangements, marital and social relationships and attitudes.

Personal lifestyles

Much research has been concerned with how physical behaviour among older people can affect health risks, including exercise (Muir Gray, 1985; McMurdo and Johnstone, 1995; Emery and Gatz, 1990; Hopkins *et al.*, 1990), diet (Kirkman, 1989), smoking (Vetter, 1989; Hess, 1991); drug use (Miller, 1991; Lindley *et al.*, 1992) and alcohol use (Green and Bridgham, 1991; Dunne and Schipperheijn, 1989). An overview of health-related behaviour among older people is provided by the Central Health Monitoring Unit (Department of Health, 1996). Each aspect of behaviour may affect several health risks; for example, exercise brings multiple benefits to health (Haskell, 1997). It can help maintain bone density and mobility, diminishing the risk of osteoporosis, falls and fractures (Department of Health, 1994; Tinetti *et al.*, 1994; King and Tinetti, 1995; Wagner *et al.*, 1994; Gibson, 1990), maintain musculoskeletal integrity (Isdale, 1993), reduce obesity and blood pressure, diminishing the risk of cardiovascular disease and stroke (Blumenthal *et al.*, 1989; WHO, 1995) and improve mental functioning (Baylor and Spirdoso, 1988; Emery and Gatz, 1990; Rogers, Meyer and Mortel, 1990). Conversely, a condition such as osteoporosis is influenced by exercise, diet and hormone replacement therapy.

Survey data on the health-related behaviour of people living in private households is provided by the Health Survey for England carried out annually since 1991 (Colhoun and Prescott-Clarke (1996). This survey covers over 3000 people aged over 65 in each year since 1993 and 600 older people in 1991 and 1992.

Table 3.1. Self-reported maximum activity level over past four weeks. Percentage of men and women, by age group, in 1994

	Men				Women			
	45–54	55–64	65–74	75+	45–54	55–64	65–74	75+
Physical activity, moderate or more	86	76	71	47	88	82	67	38
Light activity	10	14	15	25	7	9	14	17
Inactive*	4	9	13	26	4	8	17	44
	100%	100%	100%	100%	100%	100%	100%	100%
N	1127	1001	877	441	1300	1059	1120	825

* had less than one 30-minute period of moderate/vigorous exercise

Source: Colhoun and Prescott-Clarke (1996): table 6.3

The proportion of people reporting physical activity in the last four weeks, at the 'moderate' or 'vigorous' level recommended for health, declines with age. The steepest decline for men was from age 54, for women from age 64 (see Table 3.1). 'Inactivity' rose with age, but this was most common among those whose disabilities could be expected to restrict exercise.

Consumption of a wide variety of items was compared according to age group, gender and social class of the head of household in the 1994 Health Survey for England (Colhoun and Prescott-Clarke, 1996: Tables 7.6 to 7.18). This conventional measure of class has been questioned as conceptually unclear since it assigns married women's class on the basis of their husband's past occupation but single, widowed, divorced and separated women's according to their own past occupation (Arber and Ginn, 1993). Among older people, women and those in higher social classes had more healthy eating habits than men and those in lower social classes. For example, 46 per cent of men aged over 65 used sugar in tea compared with 26 per cent of women; 61 per cent of men in classes IV and V used sugar compared with 34 per cent of men in classes I and II (see Table 3.2). A similar pattern was evident for use of sugar in coffee, white rather than brown or wholemeal bread, unskimmed milk, infrequent consumption of fruit, vegetables or high-fibre cereals, routinely adding salt at table and not taking vitamin supplements.

Table 3.2. Proportion of men and women over 65 consuming each item, by social class

	Men				Women			
	I/II	IIInm	IIIm	IV/V	I/II	IIInm	IIIm	IV/V
Sugar in tea	34	42	50	61	17	27	28	34
Sugar in coffee	49	54	61	68	30	40	42	46
Whole milk	41	45	44	48	41	41	43	44
White bread	46	55	62	63	32	41	47	53
Fruit eaten rarely/never	3	3	7	9	4	5	7	5
Vegetables <1–2 days/week	3	5	6	10	4	5	5	10
Salt added routinely at table	30	33	38	37	11	14	16	18
No vitamin/mineral supplements	68	69	78	74	57	65	69	70
N	386	135	471	237	418	377	436	503

Source: Colhoun and Prescott-Clarke (1996): chapter 7

No information was reported on differences in diet according to ethnicity. Older people were slightly more likely than younger to eat white rather than other bread and less likely to use skimmed milk, but for other items their diet was at least as healthy as for younger people.

Smoking and consumption of alcohol are shown for older people in Table 3.3. Alcohol in excess of the recommended maximum weekly limit at the time of the survey (21 units for men and 14 for women) was less common among those over 65 than among younger people. In 1994, about a third of younger men but 20 per cent of men aged 65 to 74 and 12 per cent of men over 75 exceeded the limit. Among women, much lower proportions exceeded the limit, with those over 75 least likely to do so. Between 1991 and 1994, exceeding the limit became more common for women aged 65 to 74 but less common among men over 75.

Table 3.3. Change over time in self-reported behaviours among men and women aged over 65, by age group and year. Percentages with the behaviour

		Men				Women			
		1991	**1992**	**1993**	**1994**	**1991**	**1992**	**1993**	**1994**
Cigarette smoker	65–74	27	26	20	21	17	18	18	19
	75+	14	15	13	12	15	16	11	11
Alcohol intake of	65–74	20	19	20	20	4	8	9	9
over 21(14) units	75+	17	11	13	12	7	6	7	6
Activity level 0*	65–74	31	35	35	29	43	39	36	33
	75+	60	43	47	53	65	56	62	62
N	65–74	180	235	895	876	216	287	1090	1119
	75+	114	127	474	440	171	211	828	825

* on combined frequency–intensity scale

Source: Colhoun and Prescott-Clarke (1996): tables 9.4, 10.4 and 6.7

Older people are less likely than younger to be current cigarette smokers. In 1994, a fifth of those aged 65 to 74 and just over 10 per cent of those aged over 75 smoked compared with about a third of working age adults (Colhoun and Prescott-Clarke, 1996). Between 1991 and 1994, the prevalence of smoking had declined among older people, with the exception of women aged 65 to 74 who showed a very small increase (see Table 3.3). The latter reflects the tendency for successive cohorts of women to have smoking habits more similar to men's. The general decline in prevalence of smoking was due to a rising proportion who had given up smoking, rather than an increase in the proportion who had never smoked. The association of smoking with lower social class, for both men and women, is confirmed, although the reported analysis by class does not distinguish according to age group.

While the Health Surveys for England discussed above show trends over time in the health behaviour of cross-sectional samples, the Health and Lifestyle Surveys show changes in health and health behaviour of the *same* individuals over time. The 1984/5 survey (Cox *et al.*, 1987), which interviewed 9000 adults living in private households, was followed by a further survey of those who survived and could be re-interviewed seven years later in 1991/2 (Cox, Huppert and Whichelow, 1993). The 1991/2 panel included 1745 people aged over 60.

This longitudinal study confirms that heavy smokers suffer excess deterioration of respiratory function, while those who gave up between the two surveys showed some recovery towards the expected value for their age; unfortunately these results are not reported by age group

(Cox, 1993a). A substantial proportion of people aged over 60 in 1984/5 had given up smoking in the interval between the two surveys, 13 per cent of men and 9 per cent of women. Among older women, a smaller proportion had smoked in 1984/5: 21 per cent compared with 39 per cent of men (Whichelow and Cox, 1993). The decrease in smoking in the panel as a whole took place in all socioeconomic groups to much the same extent but this result was not reported for separate age groups.

There was little change in mean alcohol consumption, except for men aged 74 to 80 at the second interview, whose consumption had increased substantially (Whichelow, 1993a).

The mean body mass index (BMI) of older men and women had decreased, especially for the non-manual group, in contrast to the increase in BMI among younger people in all socioeconomic groups (Cox, 1993b). The proportion of older people above an 'acceptable' body mass index showed no increase over the interval, although the proportion of obese women (aged 67 to 80 in 1991/2) had increased slightly from 22 per cent to 26 per cent. Among men and women aged over 67 in 1991/2, a higher proportion had changed from being 'obese' to 'overweight' and from 'overweight' to 'acceptable' than in the reverse direction.

Mental state was closely related to physical health. Psychosocial health, as measured by the General Health Questionnaire (GHQ) 30 item scale, declined over the seven-year interval among those aged over 65, especially among men who had retired early and among those who had become widowed (Huppert and Whittington, 1993a). However, other research in the US suggests that adverse effects of widowhood on perceived health are neither long term nor universal (Ferraro, 1985).

The proportion of older men and women in each cohort participating in physical leisure activities had been maintained over the seven years and had even increased for some activities (Cox and Whichelow, 1993). Older people's diets showed a marked reduction in the frequency of consumption of high-fat foods by men and women in both manual and non-manual occupational groups. Use of sugar in tea and coffee had declined; however, consumption of fruit, vegetables and cereals had not increased (Whichelow, 1993b).

An aspect of behaviour largely overlooked in consideration of older people's health and health promotion is sexual activity, with its benefits (Butler and Lewis, 1976; Roberts, 1989; Kellett, 1989) and risks (Welch, 1990).

Social aspects of lifestyle

In recent years, interest in how behaviour relates to successful ageing has been extended to include the influence of social and mental aspects of behaviour in preventing cognitive decline (Baylor and Spirdoso, 1988; Emery and Gatz, 1990; Rogers, Meyer and Mortel, 1990) and improving perceived health status and longevity (Cohen and Syme, 1985; Berkman and Breslow, 1983).

There is growing evidence of the importance to health at all ages of participating actively in social networks involving family, friends and the wider community (WHO, 1992a). For example, small-scale research on older people found that they attributed their sense of wellbeing to their activities and relationships (Miller, 1991) and to 'vital involvement' (Erikson, Erikson and Kivnick, 1986) more than to diet or exercise, while another study found that overcoming loneliness helped in the healing of leg ulcers (Wise, 1986).

Social support – including companionship, practical, informational and esteem support (Cohen and Willis, 1985) – has been recognised as a valuable resource for maintaining health and wellbeing (Caplan, 1974; Cassel, 1976). Some researchers have highlighted the role of social support in protecting against clinical depression (Brown and Harris, 1978; Lowenthal and Haven, 1968), while others have claimed reductions in mortality (Berkman and Syme, 1979; Blazer, 1982). The type of supportive social network surrounding an older person is related to their degree of frailty (Wenger, 1989).

Several alternative hypotheses have been proposed to explain how social support contributes to health. The first is that social support acts as a buffer against the stresses of life, protecting the individual from the pathogenic effects of stress on health (Cohen and Willis, 1985; WHO, 1992a; Bankoff, 1983). The second is that social support improves health directly by enhancing self-esteem and the sense of security (Thoits, 1982). A third explanation is that social support encourages preventive health behaviours (Abella and Heslin, 1984; Langlie, 1977); social networks provide information and establish ways of coping with decline in health (Jerrome, 1990).

Social support may be measured in terms of the amount and frequency of social contact, and also in terms of the perceived emotional quality of the supportive relationships; these two aspects of social support may influence health in different ways (Qureshi, 1990).

Older people are particularly vulnerable to lack of social contact associated with the death or institutionalisation of partner, siblings or members of their peer group. Because of the marriage age differential and women's greater longevity, half of older women in England and Wales are widowed compared with only 17 per cent of men (OPCS, 1990: Table 7); in 1985, nearly half of women aged over 65 lived alone compared with a fifth of men (Arber and Ginn, 1991: p.172). Older widowers are more likely than widows to remarry. In 1991, the remarriage rate of widowers aged 65 to 74 was 12 per cent compared with 2 per cent for widows, while over age 75 the rates were 3 per cent for widowers and less than half a per cent for widows (Davidson, 1996). There is a consensus among researchers that women grieve while men replace their lost partner. For married men, their wife is often their confidante, whereas a close friend is more likely to perform this role for married women, so that the impact of widowhood differs for men and women (Arber and Ginn, 1991; Davidson, 1996). Older widows may face multiple barriers to rebuilding a social life (Lopata, 1973).

The greater longevity of married people has been frequently demonstrated, theorised as due to both a 'health protective' effect, in which marriage increases social networks, encourages healthy behaviour, provides informal care, increases economic resources and buffers against stress, and to the selection into marriage of healthier individuals (Goldman, Korenman and Weinstein, 1995). Research using longitudinal data on older people in the US distinguished the direct effects on health of the marital relationship from the effects of socioeconomic status and the social environment. After taking account of these factors, as well as age, ethnicity and initial health status, mortality was raised only for widowed men relative to married, not for single or widowed women (Goldman, Korenman and Weinstein, 1995). This study suggests the protection effect of marriage is more important than the selection effect and confirms the positive association of a socially active lifestyle with better health outcomes. Widowed men and women suffered a greater decline over time in functional ability than married, but single women had better health outcomes than married. This points to the importance to health of relationships other than marriage, especially for women.

Living alone restricts opportunities for social interaction, especially if mobility is limited, there is no access to private transport and public transport is poor or unaffordable. All these conditions are more common among older women than men. Older women have lower personal income than men and are less likely than men to have access to a car (Arber and Ginn, 1991). Although the health of older people living alone is similar to that of other older people, this partly reflects the selection process whereby the most frail move to live with others or into residential care. Older women living alone are a particularly vulnerable group because of the combination of a high prevalence of frailty with lack of material resources or help in the household. For these reasons, older women are twice as likely as men to live in a residential establishment (Arber and Ginn, 1991). Class and the possession of material resources also influence the ability to maintain social activities and relationships.

The Health and Lifestyle Survey of 1991/2 (Cox, Huppert and Whichelow, 1993) confirms that among those aged over 67, high malaise is more likely for those living alone, and is more common among older women than men (Swain, 1993b). Adverse life events experienced by older people were associated with the development of ill health, including not only depression but physical conditions (Cox, Huppert and Whichelow, 1993). Older people reported less stress than younger and men less than women (Whittington and Huppert, 1993). Older men and women whose roles and attachments had decreased between 1984/5 and 1991/2 were most likely to have increased malaise; health was less likely to be assessed positively at the second interview for all older people except those whose roles and attachments had increased between the two surveys (Swain, 1993b).

The quality as well as the quantity of relationships is relevant to older people's morale, confirming the finding by Brown and Harris (1978) among younger people. Research by Murphy (1982) with older Londoners found a confiding relationship protected against depression. Marriage is often the main source of such a relationship but as we have seen this is less available to older women than men.

For those who live alone, personal friendships are often the main source of emotional support, enduring when the roles of worker and spouse have been lost (Atchley, 1980; Jerrome, 1981; Crohan and Antonucci, 1989). Older women tend to have better-developed skills than men in making close friends, due to a lifetime of 'relationship work'. Based on reciprocity and mutual interests, friendships affirm identity and self-worth in a way that relationships with extended families may not (Crohan and Antonucci, 1989). Opportunities for close friendship are socially structured (Allan and Adams, 1989), being dependent on the amount of 'personal space' (Deem, 1982) in which personal life can be developed. Thus close and satisfying relationships promote health but tend to be less available to older people who are most constrained by ill health and disability, especially if material resources are also lacking.

Where older people have become frail and in need of care, practical and emotional support is primarily provided by kin. Over a third of the total time spent on practical informal care to older people is supplied by other older people, mainly spouses (Arber and Ginn, 1990). Concern has been expressed that informal care provided by younger kin will decline due to their geographical migration and increased employment of women (WHO, 1993; Dooghe, 1992). Yet there is no evidence that employed women are less likely than the non-employed to provide care for parents/in-law, although caring does constrain carers' employment, earnings, social life and health (Arber and Ginn, 1995a; Martin Matthews and Campbell, 1995).

Mental abilities are clearly important both for maintaining social relationships and for adequate self-care. Cognitive functions, measured in the two Health and Lifestyle Surveys (Cox, Huppert and Whichelow, 1993) were better in younger than older people, due to both age and cohort effects. Later cohorts' better scores were associated with more education, lending some support to the 'use it or lose it' hypothesis (Orrell and Sahakin, 1995); but within each cohort performance on several measures, including memory, declined with age after age 60. There was some evidence that women's age-related decline in mental function began later than men's (Huppert and Whittington, 1993b).

Senile dementia is a major cause of disability and the most common cause of older people's admission to mental illness hospitals, followed by psychoses and depression (DHSS, 1989). Although the outlook for prevention is unpromising, there has been interest in the possibility that continuing mental activity prevents or slows decline (Orrell and Sahakin, 1995; Perrson and Skoog, 1996), and there may be scope for improved management of symptoms. Moreover, senile dementia (including Alzheimer's Disease) may sometimes be misdiagnosed in older people suffering from treatable depression (Sidell, 1995; Macdonald, 1986).

Attitudes to behaviour and health

Attitudes to health affect whether health promotion messages result in more healthy lifestyles (Downie, Fyfe and Tannahill, 1992). These authors provide a comprehensive account of the factors influencing changes in attitudes and behaviour. The majority of people reject a fatalistic attitude to health, believing they can influence their chance of illness, but older people are more likely than younger to think health is a matter of luck: in the British Social Attitudes Survey, this was the view of 23 per cent of people aged over 55 compared with 11 per cent of 35- to 54-year-olds (Jowell, Witherspoon and Brook, 1990). Among people of all ages there was no gender difference, but fatalistic attitudes were more common among those in manual classes and lacking educational qualifications.

Since early detection and treatment of diseases, especially cancers, is vital in preventing or limiting the development of disease, willingness and ability to report symptoms at an early stage and (among women) to seek breast and cervical screening are an important aspect of health behaviour. Research in the US has highlighted the effect of poverty among older non-married women in delaying seeking health care, an issue which, as yet, is less relevant in Britain (Keith, 1987).

Results from the Health and Lifestyle Surveys (Cox, Huppert and Whichelow, 1993) are consistent with these attitudinal differences according to age and class. Reports of changing diet were less common among those aged over 60 at first interview than among those aged under 60, 37 per cent compared with 59 per cent. Whereas younger people most often attributed a change in behaviour to health campaigns, the most common reason given by older people was illness (Whichelow, 1993b). Nevertheless, older people demonstrated an increase over time in both awareness of, and participation in, health-promoting behaviour (Swain, 1993a). Older people in non-manual occupational groups were more likely than those in manual groups to report adopting healthy behaviours in order to improve their health (Swain, 1993b).

Summary

In some aspects of behaviour, such as smoking and drinking, older people's lifestyle is healthier than that of younger people, while in terms of diet there is little difference according to age. Not surprisingly, older people's physical activity is less than that of younger people, and is lowest among older women. Diets are more health-oriented among older women than men and among those in a non-manual occupational group.

Longitudinal research shows that older people have modified their behaviour in terms of smoking, alcohol, exercise and type of diet. A decline in psychosocial health is likely to stem from loss of supportive social roles and relationships, as in widowhood. Widows are a particularly vulnerable group, lacking either the social, caring and financial resources of married women or the supportive social networks built up by single women.

Unfortunately, although the health surveys outlined show gender and age group differences in older people's health behaviour, little is reported on how their lifestyle varies with socioeconomic position.

While the evidence of lifestyle change among older people indicates that the risk of cardiovascular disease, stroke, certain cancers, cirrhosis and fractures will decline, it is less clear that the incidence and impact of other common and distressing conditions of later life, such as arthritis, impaired hearing or vision and Alzheimer's Disease, can be reduced by behavioural change. Some writers have pointed out the danger that a culture of health promotion centred mainly on individual behavioural change may lead to older people being blamed for their illness (Nettleton, 1996; Sidell, 1995). Many of the causes of ill health are outside the individual's control, including the socioeconomic factors outlined in Chapter 2 and the nature of the local community, as discussed in Chapter 4.

Chapter 4

OLDER PEOPLE'S HEALTH AND THE LOCAL ENVIRONMENT

Chapters 2 and 3 considered influences at the macro level and at the household, or individual, level on older people's health. Although there is evidence of variations in health according to locality of residence, less research attention has been paid to how the quality of the local environment may affect the health of older people (Wallace, 1994). In this chapter, we consider how the physical environment, infrastructural services and the social environment may affect the health of older people and the potential for local authorities and health professionals to improve the local environment.

The hazards to health in the physical environment, outlined in WHO (1993), interact with individual risk factors, contributing to cancer, cardiovascular diseases, respiratory disorders, allergies, neurological and motor disorders and accidental injuries. The physical environment includes the extent of chemical and noise pollution from traffic and industry, design and adequacy of housing, access to wholesome water and food. Although a poor environment affects health at all ages, the effects of respiratory disorders from air pollution and enteric diseases from microbiological contamination of food or water are likely to be more serious for older people than for the rest of the population. Moreover, the cumulative risks to health will be greatest for older people. The quality of indoor air also affects health (WHO, 1992b) and this, along with adequate heating to prevent hypothermia (OPCS, 1986; Collins, 1986; McManus, 1985; Roberts and Boardman, 1989), is especially important to housebound older people. Traffic and poorly maintained pavements present a greater risk of accidents to older than to younger adults because they are more likely to have failing eyesight, poor balance, low muscle strength and dizziness. The domination of local environments by a car culture is especially hostile to the health of children and older people.

A number of public health measures are proposed by WHO at national, regional and local level: environmental health monitoring and enforcement, local authority action to pedestrianise, to reduce noise and fumes, to design the built environment so as to promote safety and a sense of belonging, to encourage exercise and social interaction through providing parks and recreational facilities (WHO, 1993: p.111), and to encourage maintenance of local facilities such as shops, clubs, clinics and so on which do not require long journeys.

Infrastructural services include GPs, hospitals, health visitors, local authority social services, leisure and education facilities and public transport. Adequate and appropriate local health services are important to older people's physical health and also to their morale. An ageist portrayal of older people as a 'burden' on the NHS may be reinforced by ageism in medical practice (French, 1990; Henwood, 1990). The quality of communication between patient and doctor is vital to effective health care (Downie, Fyfe and Tannahill, 1992), and this is especially so for older people (Beisecker and Thompson, 1995). Approachability of GPs, willingness to give time to a patient, to appreciate their own perspective and to make home visits may be especially important to older people.

If doctors dismiss aches and pains as 'due to old age', this may inhibit older people from reporting symptoms, leading to delay in treatment. Ageism in screening programmes, exemplified by the exclusion of women over 65 from routine screening for breast and cervical cancer, delays discovery of disease (Henwood, 1990); 40 per cent of deaths from cervical cancer occur in women aged over 65. Because of the exclusion of older people from clinical trials of drug dosages (MRC, 1994) and lack of appreciation of the effects of ageing on response to drugs, the effects of prescribed drugs are less predictable and can be iatrogenic: 'Adverse reactions to drugs comprise a significant problem in the care of the elderly' (Miller, 1991).

For ethnic minority elders, health services (Glendenning, 1990) and social services (Bowling, 1990; Hill, 1990; Tarpey, 1990) are not always sensitive to their needs. The social devaluation associated with ageing is compounded by racism (Norman, 1985) and older people from ethnic minorities tend to be poorer than whites (Raleigh, 1992). They face greater difficulties in obtaining health care, housing and social services (Morton, 1993), due to the assumption that families are available to help, lack of information and ethnocentric provision (Fennell, Phillipson and Evers, 1988). Preference for integrated or special services differs according to ethnic group (Askham, Henshaw and Tarpey, 1993).

Several reforms to the NHS since the 1980s are likely to bear harder on older than younger people. Fundholding arrangements provide an incentive to GPs to minimise the number of people with poor health in their practice. Hospital trusts' increasing drive to maximise patient turnover may lead to premature discharge of older people if account is not taken of their longer time to recover from illness and surgical procedures. Early discharge is likely to prejudice the chance of full rehabilitation, especially where there is poor coordination with social services in arranging for care at home (Age Concern, 1995). Rational-isation of hospital provision, with closure of local units, increases the difficulty of attending for those lacking private transport; among those aged over 65, just over half of men have access to a car and less than a third of women (Arber and Ginn, 1991).

The reforms in social services provision since the 1990 NHS and Community Care Act have brought stricter rationing and increased charges for home care services to older people. A survey of social services departments found that nearly three-quarters of older people who before 1993 would have received statutory domiciliary services no longer receive any (AMA and ACC, 1995). Local authorities have been compelled to increase charges for home care and respite care, although charging policy has been varied (AMA, 1994). The danger is that fear of being unable to pay charges may deter older people from seeking the care they need, with adverse effects on their health and wellbeing. Cuts in day centres and lunch clubs for older people, or in transport provid-ed by social services departments to enable attendance, reduce the opportunities for older people to maintain social activities. Older women have suffered particularly acutely from all these developments because of their lower income, greater disability and higher likelihood of living alone (see Chapter 2 and Arber and Ginn, 1991). Home care staff and day centre staff have a valuable role in monitoring older peo-ple's health and alerting relatives or appropriate medical staff when appropriate. They also provide a potential channel for health educa-tion, in conjunction with health care professionals.

Recreational and educational facilities, especially if affordable, easi-ly accessible and meeting the preferences of older people, can have health benefits beyond their ostensible purpose (Gray, 1986). For exam-ple, music and movement exercises can build confidence and provide opportunities for sociability and companionship (Morris, 1986).

The quality of the local social environment is less easy to define than in the case of the physical environment. It includes such factors as actu-al and perceived safety, stability, extensiveness and overlapping of social networks and degree of trust and neighbourliness. Giddens (1994) argues that ontological security – a sense of continuity, order, trust and belonging – provides the foundation for a person's confidence and self-identity. In Chapter 2, the association of social activities with health and wellbeing was noted. A primary concern of older people is that they can feel safe; fear of attack in the street, especially after dark if street lighting is poor, makes it hard to maintain social and leisure activ-ities. Aspects of the social environment likely to enhance older people's wellbeing include knowing and trusting their neighbours and feeling integrated and valued in the community. Studies in the US found that devout religiousness among older people protected them against depression and enhanced health (Koenig, 1991; 1993), while those involved with a religious community had a more positive outlook and better functional abilities than other older people (Idler and Kasl, 1992). Desire for sociability with neighbours varies, but confidence in the goodwill of nearby residents is likely to promote a sense of security and belonging, especially for those older people who live alone and have no local kin. Predictors of residential satisfaction among older women living alone in the US are considered by Carp and Christensen (1986). Although many older people already work in voluntary organisations, expanding older people's opportunities to contribute as volunteers, for example in primary schools or in health and caring services, could maintain the social integration and sense of purpose important to health. Local authorities can facilitate self-help and mutual aid projects among older people, for example to cope with bereavement (Silverman, 1986). Improving such intangibles as social integration is no easy task for local authorities and health professionals, especially where national policies have contributed to socially disruptive trends.

Local action to improve older people's health would need to encompass both the quality of the local environment, health and screening services, and the development of health education/promotion programmes focused on individuals' lifestyles (Gray, 1985). A wide range of screening programmes for older people has been recommended by US experts (Beers, Fink and Beck, 1991). Local health education programmes with older people have been found to be an important complement to the use of national media (Tones, 1981). A number of health promotion projects and plans, initiated by statutory bodies, GPs and voluntary organisations, are outlined by Dalley *et al.* (1996).

Approaches to health education range from the traditional to the 'modern' (Downie, Fyfe and Tannahill, 1992). The traditional, or 'top down' approach, based on a model of the rational individual, involves medical educators providing information on preventing ill health to a target group, neglecting the social determinants of health. A 'modern' approach aims to promote positive health and is more collaborative and egalitarian, helping participants to clarify their own values, acquire lifeskills and develop self-esteem.

Given the diversity of older people in terms of their gender, social class, ethnicity, functional abilities and preferences, wide consultation with older people is needed to ensure a suitable range of programmes. These could include health education, physical fitness, adult education, social activities and leisure pursuits. They would need to be accessible to those with impaired mobility, vision, hearing or with very limited income and to be responsive to the needs of ethnic minority elders. For example, encouraging use of leisure and exercise facilities by Asian elders (especially women) requires understanding cultural barriers (Hounslow Leisure Services, 1997). Programmes need to extend into residential and nursing homes and to be monitored and reviewed.

A partnership in which local authority departments and health professionals cooperate with local pensioners' organisations and Older People's Forums (Thornton and Tozer, 1994; Carter and Nash, 1992) in planning and implementing programmes will help ensure diverse needs are met. Locally-based 'Ageing Well' pilot projects, launched in 1993 in the UK, explore the potential of 'Senior Health Mentors' (trained older volunteers) in working with older people to encourage healthy lifestyles (Ageing Well Europe, 1996; Freeman, 1994; Wright, 1997). Such schemes point the way to a fruitful partnership between the statutory and voluntary sectors, although it is too early for a full evaluation.

Summary

The influence of the local physical, social and infrastructural environment on older people's health has been little researched. In health care, ageist assumptions and practices have been detrimental to older people's health in several ways, ranging from the cuts in continuing care beds in hospitals to lack of knowledge of how age affects the response to prescribed medicines. Scope for action by local authorities to improve older people's health include reducing local physical hazards to health; ensuring availability and affordability of domiciliary social services, day centres, educational, social and leisure facilities; fostering a positive social environment; and providing health education and promotion programmes designed in consultation with older people.

Although much could be done by local authorities, if sufficient resources were made available, to promote older people's health and quality of life, local efforts need to be complemented by national policies to facilitate healthy behaviour in a healthy environment (Downie, Fyfe and Tannahill, 1992). A ban on tobacco advertising would end the anomaly in which health education messages compete with contrary persuasion from advertisements. More could be done at national level, including banning advertising of tobacco products, enforcing safety regulations in food processing and retailing, controlling factory effluents, improving standards in housing, facilitating public instead of private transport and, above all, to raise the standard of living of older people. As a Swedish report argues, 'Adaptation of the social environment to the abilities and needs of elderly people is seen as the major health promotion strategy for adding years to life' (Levi and Cox, 1994: p.336).

The four chapters in Part II discuss alternative methods of researching health and health promotion issues among older people.

Part II

Researching older people's health promotion

Chapter 5

POTENTIAL OF SECONDARY ANALYSIS OF EXISTING DATA

The secondary analysis of existing survey data has an increasingly important role in social research. This method is more cost-effective than initiating new survey research and can be less time-consuming when quick results are needed (Hakim, 1982; Dale, Arber and Procter, 1988).

The variety of national datasets available provides an extensive and unique resource of information, most of which are under-analysed in the original published reports. Large-scale surveys benefit from the resources needed to collect high quality data from a large and representative sample. This means that the conclusions drawn from a study focused on older people can be generalised and the results compared with the population as a whole. Many social surveys consistently use standardised summary measures for key concepts such as social class or ethnic background and can therefore be used as complementary sources of data or to replicate previous findings.

This chapter discusses the analytic potential and limitations of the following datasets for the study of older people's health and health promotion needs: the Health Education Monitoring Survey (HEMS), the Health and Lifestyles Survey 1984/5 and 1991/2 (HALS), the Health and Lifestyle Survey of the UK population, the Health Survey for England 1991–6 (HSE) and the General Household Survey (GHS). Further details about the topics covered in each survey are included in the Appendix. All these datasets allow for a cross-sectional analysis of the population. One limitation of cross-sectional analysis is that any claims about the *direction of causality* between health states, personal characteristics and behaviour may be problematic due to possible health selection effects. This issue is discussed further in Chapter 8.

Health Education and Monitoring Survey 1995

The main aim of the Health Education and Monitoring Survey (HEMS) was to examine health-related knowledge, attitudes and behaviour, with reference to the progress being made towards Health of the Nation targets (Bridgwood *et al.*, 1996). The sample was restricted to adults aged between 16 and 74 years living in private households in England.

A probability sample was taken from the Postcode Address File of approximately 5000 adults aged between 16 and 74 years, with an overall response rate of 76 per cent. Within each eligible household, one adult resident was interviewed at random in 1995. Approximately 30 per cent of the total sample are aged between 55 and 74 years, of which 646 are male and 775 female.

The key topics covered by the questionnaire include coronary heart disease and cancer, along with the health consequences associated with smoking, drinking, diet and blood pressure. (Older people aged 54–74 years are excluded from the section on sexual health.) Many questions in these sections relate to health attitudes and beliefs about disease prevention and their own health status. These questions could form the basis of a factor analysis which would serve to highlight the different components or 'factors' underlying beliefs about health-promoting or health-damaging behaviour. These derived factors can then be used as explanatory variables for further secondary analysis (Procter, 1993).

The morbidity indicators included in the survey are self-reported long-standing illness (LI), limiting long-standing illness (LLI) and general health, but specific information on mental health is lacking. The importance of health beliefs and knowledge in determining actual (physical) health status can thus be examined. Information obtained about number of GP consultations in the last year allows older people's utilisation of this service to be examined and related to their health status. However, information about inpatient or outpatient hospital attendances is not included.

The survey also contains measures of socioeconomic status, such as occupational social class and educational level, as well as indicators of material deprivation, namely housing tenure and car ownership. The relationship between socioeconomic background and health status can be investigated to illuminate health inequalities. The effect of socioeconomic status on health and health behaviours may vary across the 54- to 74-year-old age group, due to factors such as widowhood and leaving the workforce. The dataset contains information about marital status and employment status, making it possible to identify the retired, the widowed and those living alone or with others.

In addition to socioeconomic status, information about ethnic origin is obtained through a self-assessment measure. Ethnicity could be an important determinant of health status and behaviour. However, the number of older people classified as ethnic minority in this study is very small due to the overall sample size and the younger age structure of these ethnic populations.

Health and Lifestyles Survey 1984/5 and 1991/2

The Health and Lifestyle Survey (HALS) covers a national sample of adults living in private households in England, Wales and Scotland. Addresses were selected randomly from the electoral register and one resident aged 18 years or above was interviewed in every household, giving a total sample size of 9003 in 1984/5. No upper age limit was applied; approximately 3700 respondents are aged over 50 years and 6 per cent of males and 9 per cent of females are aged over 75 years. The survey includes a self-completion questionnaire assessing personality and psychiatric status and also physiological measurements such as height, weight and blood pressure.

The inclusion of data assessing mental health, cognitive functioning and psychiatric status is the main strength of this survey, with few other surveys based upon such a representative sample. However, it is important to be aware that a differential non-response rate may affect the very elderly population, with the self-completion and physical measurement sections more likely to be completed by those with greater mental and physical capabilities (Blaxter, 1990).

Compared to HEMS, the Health and Lifestyle Survey is able to view health as a multi-dimensional concept, incorporating self-reports of morbidity along with more 'objective' cognitive tests and possible psycho-social factors such as family contact and perceived social support. The consideration of mental health and psycho-social factors is particularly relevant to the study of an ageing population. The data enable cognitive functioning to be examined in the 'healthy' older population as well as those classified as having a long-standing limiting illness or an adverse lifestyle. Respondents who report a long-standing limiting illness are asked about how this has limited their ability to perform a range of tasks. Using these questions it would be possible to construct some sort of 'disability index' for older people that would distinguish different levels of infirmity (Arber and Ginn 1993). This index could then be related to the individual's lifestyle or mental health. Unfortunately the survey does not contain complementary data about any informal care received by disabled older people.

All older people are asked questions that relate to exercise, work and leisure. These data can be used to classify levels of activity and inactivity amongst older people and the implications for health status and lifestyle can be considered. Detailed questions also exist about drinking, smoking and nutrition that include some retrospective information, for example, alcohol consumption in the last week. However, the demand on memory may make these data less suitable for very old people included in the sample.

As with HEMS, the survey contains information about the health knowledge, beliefs and intentions of respondents. Supplementing the information about psycho-social factors discussed earlier are direct questions about living circumstances that are perceived to affect health status, such as housing, level of income and relationships. This information can be related to actual measures of socioeconomic status and health status. Unlike the previous survey, HALS contains information about the employment status of a spouse/partner and also the length of time an individual has been widowed. These variables may have implications for individual health status and socioeconomic position.

The dataset does not contain information about the number of doctor consultations or hospital visits; therefore the use of these services cannot be studied. However, information is included about the receipt of prescriptions, the type of health complaint experienced and whether this has been treated by a doctor or hospital. By examining the frequency and range of health problems between the two HALS surveys and relating this to individual lifestyle, it may be possible to examine the 'compression of morbidity' argument that the third age is associated with longer active life and shorter periods of ill health and disability (Fries, 1980; 1989).

The data collected on ethnic origin rely upon the assessment of the interviewer and are coded once the interview has been completed. This is unfortunate because the coding categories used are much more general and imprecise than individual self-assessment. However, the larger sample size on which this survey is based would allow some analysis of variations in health by ethnic origin.

A Health and Lifestyle follow-up survey was completed in 1991/2. Figures show that a total of 2417 respondents in this sample are aged 53+ years, of which 56 per cent are female and 44 per cent male (Cox, Huppert and Whichelow, 1993). Included in this survey are respondents who have moved into residential care. Information about cause of death continues to be added to the database. The potential of using the HALS data for longitudinal analysis is examined in Chapter 8.

Health and Lifestyle Survey of the UK population

This survey was commissioned by the Health Education Authority and conducted by MORI in 1992 (HEA, 1995) to assess health needs and the factors contributing to health status. A probability sample of 5000 people aged between 16 and 74 years was used, based on private households in England, Scotland, Wales and Northern Ireland. The sample structure allowed for 4000 interviews with 16- to 54-year-olds and 1000 with respondents aged 55–74 years. A self-completion questionnaire on sexual health was not given to this older age group. All data were weighted in proportion with household size, age, sex, and the 1992 population projections for each country.

Unlike the previous two surveys, the MORI dataset contains detailed information about ethnic background, with additional questions on religion and country of birth. Unfortunately, because of the small size of the older age sample, it would not be possible to analyse ethnic patterning in health status and beliefs.

The health indicators included in the survey are self-reported long-standing illness and limiting long-standing illness. A section also exists about psycho-social health, where respondents report the degree of stress associated with life events, such as retirement, financial difficulties and moving house – all of which are relevant to older people. Stress can also be related to lifestyle as respondents are asked about 'coping strategies' they may deploy when under stress, such as smoking, drinking or obtaining a medical prescription.

Unlike the previous two surveys, health perceptions are located within the context of the environment, workplace and family home. It is possible to relate these health attitudes and beliefs to socioeconomic background as variables such as housing tenure, accommodation type and car ownership are included.

A large section of the survey focuses on the quality of visits to the general practitioner surgery. Unlike most surveys, this measures individual perceptions of the consultation with the doctor, nurse or receptionist and gives an indicator of waiting time, travel to the surgery and the reason for consulting the doctor. Attitudinal information about the convenience and usefulness of the surgery visit is an uncommon feature of large-scale surveys and the information could be used to examine older people's utilisation of this service.

Health Survey for England

The Health Survey for England (HSE) is a continuous annual survey of private households that began in 1991 to monitor changes in the nation's health with reference to the Health of the Nation target areas. A random sample of addresses was selected from the Postcode Address File using a multi-stage sample design (Breeze, Trevor and Wilmot, 1994). Unlike the previous datasets discussed, all adults in the household aged 16 or above were included in the survey. Each Health

Survey consists of three main elements: the interview, a self-completion questionnaire on psycho-social health and the taking of physiological measurements, including a blood sample. The non-response rate therefore varies across these three elements of the survey design, with fewer physical measurements recorded for older people due to physical impairment (Bennett *et al.*, 1995).

In 1991 and 1992 the overall sample size of the Health Survey is much smaller than subsequent years, being 3242 and 4018 respectively. Approximately 9 per cent of individuals included in each of these years are over the age of 75 (White *et al.*, 1993; Breeze *et al.*, 1994). From 1993 onwards, data are collected continuously throughout the year with a much larger sample size of approximately 16,000 each year. In 1993 a total of 5502 individuals are aged 55+ years, of which approximately 24 per cent are over 74 years. For the purposes of analysis, several different years of the Health Survey can be combined in order to produce a larger sample from which more reliable estimates and generalisations can be made about older people's health and health behaviour.

The first four Health Surveys, from 1991 to 1994, focus upon cardiovascular disease (CVD) as a major cause of morbidity, and examine in detail the associated risk factors such as diet, exercise and smoking. The questionnaire focuses on a detailed symptomology of chest pain that can be differentiated in terms of severity. To supplement this self-reported information, physical measurements are taken. Blood pressure is measured and height and weight measurements are used to calculate a body mass index. A blood sample is tested for signs of diabetes and clotting rate. All respondents are questioned about their use of general practitioner services, but only those reporting CVD are asked about hospital visits within the last year. Information about the nature of the doctor consultation or any referrals made by a doctor to a hospital service is not included. However, all prescribed medicines are recorded and classified into pharmacological groups for analysis. This emphasis of the health survey data on detailed 'factual' information means that attitudinal information is rarely included.

Diet and nutrition forms a main topic area in 1993 and 1994 that allows 'unhealthy diets' to be identified, such as those high in salt or fat, which can be related to health status. Questions also exist about levels of physical activity and exercise within a four-week period, focusing on activities such as gardening and housework which may be more relevant to older people than measures of formal sporting activity. Further information about health behaviours such as smoking and drinking includes both current and past behaviour, thus distinguishing between ex-smokers and non-smokers. Within the section on alcohol consumption, all respondents are asked to complete a frequency list that estimates the alcohol consumed within the last year. Although a detailed source of information, this may prove more unreliable for older respondents due to memory difficulties.

The most recent Health Surveys for 1995 and 1996 change their focus from CVD to asthma and related respiratory conditions, considering symptoms and medications in detail. The 1995 Health Survey contains a section on disability that is most relevant to the older population. Respondents are questioned on their ability to perform a range of tasks, such as walking up stairs or getting out of bed unaided. As previously mentioned in the discussion on the Health and Lifestyle Survey (HALS), this information could be used to produce a scale of disability that reflects the degree of mobility amongst older people. Unlike HALS, this disability information is collected for all older respondents, not just those reporting a long-standing illness or disability.

In both 1995 and 1996, questions are included on accident morbidity that covers how and why the accident happened and what intervention (if any) was sought as a result. The survey enables the occurrence of these accidents to be related to both living circumstances, such as whether the respondent lives alone or with others, and personal circumstances such as health status and disability.

All respondents are asked to fill in a self-completion questionnaire on psycho-social health that includes the General Health Questionnaire 12-item scale. This scale measures psychiatric symptoms such as depression, anxiety and social functioning. The results from this scale can be used to investigate the relationship between psychiatric illness and physical illness or health behaviours. Also included in each year of the survey is core information that relates to socioeconomic background, such as housing tenure, car availability, employment and educational level. Information about ethnic origin is obtained by a self-assessment question. The large sample size of the Health Survey makes any analysis using ethnic origin more reliable.

British General Household Survey

The General Household Survey (GHS) is a multi-purpose continuous survey that has been conducted annually by the government since 1971. It provides a nationally representative sample of approximately 10,000 private households in Great Britain each year (Bennett *et al.*, 1996). Since 1984 these households have been selected from the Postcode Address File (previously the Electoral Register was used). The addresses are then stratified according to key housing and economic indicators that are contained in the Census at postcode sector level. At each household, all adults aged 16+ years are interviewed, with proxy interviews being conducted where this is not possible, approximately 25,000 interviews per year. A response rate of 80–82 per cent is typically obtained each year. The resulting dataset has a hierarchical structure, with information available for analysis at the level of the household, family, individual and individual's behaviour (Dale, Arber and Procter, 1988). The complex structure of the GHS allows the secondary analyst to link information from different individuals, such as husbands and wives, in order to analyse their characteristics.

Health has always formed a main topic area of the GHS and the large sample size of the survey makes it an extremely powerful data source with which to analyse the health of older people. The proportion of the sample aged over 65 years has remained consistently above 12 per cent since 1980 and among men over 65 the proportion aged over 85 has doubled from 3 to 6 per cent during this period (Goddard and Savage, 1994).

The health measures included in the General Household Survey are self-reported measures of long-standing illness, limiting long-standing illness, general health and acute illness (measured by activity being restricted due to illness in the two weeks preceding interview). Information is also obtained about hospital and general practitioner visits, with additional data about GP referrals being available for selected years of the survey. This can be used to examine utilisation of the health service by the older population, particularly with reference to their individual health status. Detailed information on smoking and drinking is included in the GHS every two years.

The broad content of the GHS enables these health data to be related to detailed information in areas such as income, household composition and socioeconomic background. Out of all the surveys considered in this chapter, the GHS has the best potential for a study of ethnic patterning in older people's health status, behaviour and utilisation. As with the HSE, several years of the GHS can be combined to provide a sufficiently large sample size for analysis. However, unlike surveys such as HALS, no questions are used to explicitly assess mental health, attitudes to health or access to health care services. The GHS also does not include any physiological measurement of health.

For the years 1980, 1985, 1991 and 1994, the GHS contains more detailed questions focused on people aged 65 and over. This provides a valuable source of information about the ability of older people to live independently in their own home, their social contacts, any visual or hearing impairments and their use of health services. The disability questions are essentially similar to those contained in the Health and Lifestyle Survey (HALS) and the Health Survey for England (HSE). However, the GHS covers a wider range of activities that may be impaired, ranging from physical mobility (such as climbing stairs) to more minor tasks such as making tea or brushing hair. A comprehensive 'disability index' can therefore be constructed which is based on a much larger sample size than the HALS. For those respondents who report that they are unable to perform a task unaided, the GHS records who usually provides help, enabling assessment of the extent to which informal care is provided by individuals within or outside the household. The 1985 survey also identifies the contribution made by informal carers which may permit some older people to remain living in their own home (Arber and Ginn, 1991).

Other data sources

The British Household Panel Survey (BHPS) is a relatively new annual survey carried out by the ESRC Research Centre for Micro-social Change at the University of Essex (Buck *et al.*, 1994). The BHPS contains information at a household and individual level and is based on a stratified sample drawn from the Postcode Address File of approximately 5000 private households in Great Britain, first interviewed in 1991. The panel design of this survey means that the same individuals are re-interviewed annually, even if they move to a new address. For each wave of the survey, the proportion of the sample aged over 65 years remains consistently above 20 per cent. Health and Caring are main topic areas and are designed to be relevant to the key issues in the Health of the Nation report (Department of Health, 1992). Data are collected on general health, the use of primary health care and aspects of health behaviour. As with the Health Survey for England, the BHPS also asks respondents to complete the General Health Questionnaire 12-item scale to assess psycho-social health. The main strength of this panel survey is the potential to analyse health changes over time. This issue is considered in more detail in Chapter 8.

A more specialised survey focused on the older population is the National Diet and Nutritional Survey of British Adults aged 65+ years (DOH/MAFF, 1997) commissioned jointly by the Department of Health and the Ministry of Agriculture, Fisheries and Food (MAFF). Unlike any of the previous surveys, the sample includes 400 respondents living in communal establishments as well as information from older people living in 1250 private households in Great Britain. Detailed information about dietary behaviour is obtained and physical samples of blood and urine are examined. The survey includes variables such as ethnic origin, employment and educational level which permit an analysis of dietary behaviour by demographic characteristics and socioeconomic background.

The Omnibus Survey is a continuous survey that has been conducted by the Office for National Statistics on a monthly basis since October 1990 (Bowling, 1995). It contains interviews with approximately 2000 adults aged over 16 years living in Great Britain each month. Although the number of older people in the sample will be limited, each month contains core information about demographic status supplemented by detailed topic information that varies from month to month. Topic areas covered include health status, disability and activity/exercise, all of which are relevant to a study of older people.

The Allied Dunbar National Fitness Survey (1990) measured physical activity and fitness levels of a random sample ($N = 4316$) of the adult population living in England. This survey includes a physical fitness appraisal for all respondents (although more limited measures are taken for those aged over 75 years). The relationship between fitness, health and wellbeing can be investigated. The main report for this survey (Activity and Health Research, 1992) did not analyse data for individuals aged over 75 years.

Summary

This chapter illustrates the range and diversity of survey data available for secondary analysis. The largest datasets, namely the General Household Survey (GHS) and the Health Survey for England (HSE) permit a full analysis of the health of the older population that can be related to a wide range of social and economic indicators. These surveys do not contain detailed attitudinal information, but these data are available in surveys such as the Health Education and Monitoring Survey (HEMS) and the Health and Lifestyle Survey of the UK population (HALS). All of the surveys discussed share common elements and can be used to complement each other in a more comprehensive analysis of the health of this older age group.

The Health and Education Monitoring Survey should be considered for further secondary analysis. However such analysis will be limited because older people aged 75+ are excluded from the sample. Any conclusions must therefore only apply to the 50- to 74-year-old age group, within which it may not be possible to perform a detailed age analysis due to the relatively small sample size. Similarly the smaller social surveys such as the Health and Lifestyle Survey of the UK population (MORI) are limited in scope for secondary analysis. The small numbers of older people would make a detailed investigation of this sub-group unreliable. The most comprehensive analysis of older people would be based on the General Household Survey which includes all older people but, as with most of the surveys discussed, it excludes those living in institutional care, who may be expected to have a poorer overall health status. The Health Survey for England has the greatest potential for secondary analysis because of the large sample of people aged over 50 and detailed questions on exercise, leisure activities, diet, smoking and drinking. Measurements of obesity and blood pressure, with blood tests for various risk factors, allows self-assessed health to be compared with clinical measures.

Chapter 6

QUALITATIVE RESEARCH ON OLDER PEOPLE'S HEALTH

While survey questions have the advantage of providing information which can be nationally representative, they are less useful in discovering salient issues and subjective meanings held by people. In order to understand how older people define health, what their priorities are for improving their quality of life and how they perceive issues around health promotion, qualitative research is of greater value. By allowing issues and perspectives to emerge from the respondents, qualitative research helps to avoid preconceptions being imposed by the researchers. For example, avoiding cultural assumptions is of particular importance in researching ethnic minorities (Stanfield, 1993).

Qualitative methods, including in-depth (that is, unstructured, or focused) interviews and focus group discussions, have been widely used in research, either to complement survey data or to inform the design of a survey. Such methods aim to 'elicit rich, detailed materials . . . [and] . . . to find out what kinds of things are happening' (Lofland, 1971: p.6). A strength of qualitative methods is the scope for probing for a fuller response on a new or particularly interesting idea expressed by respondents and in drawing out underlying beliefs rather than superficial answers. In qualitative research, it is especially important to ensure that respondents are respected and valued for their contribution. In this chapter, we consider how in-depth interviews and focus groups could be used in researching older people's health needs and health promotion.

In-depth interviews

In-depth interviews are mainly used to identify the most salient dimensions of a topic; to establish the range of opinion on an issue; to discover the concepts, language and reasoning used by respondents; and to form tentative hypotheses about the motivation underlying behaviour and attitudes. This type of interview is a common means of recording very detailed data such as a life history, or material which is complex or sensitive (Fielding, 1993). Because of its adaptability and personalised nature, the method is particularly suitable for use with frail or older individuals.

In contrast to the structured interview used in surveys, an in-depth interview allows a great deal of flexibility in the content and flow of the interview. Interviewers have an 'interview guide' which lists topics they want the respondent to talk about but they are free to phrase and order the questions so as to be sensitive to what the respondent has to say. The method gives respondents a voice, allowing them to define the issues relevant to them. The exchange, which resembles a 'guided conversation', is tape recorded for later transcription and can be analysed using a range of software-assisted techniques.

We would recommend focused interviews with 60 older people living in the community and a similar number living in a residential setting. The interviewed sample would need to ensure an adequate range of individuals in terms of age, gender, social class and ethnicity, as well as including individuals with chronic illnesses and disabilities. Interviewing older people living in an institutional setting as well as those living in the community would enable comparison of the experiences and attitudes of those with similar functional abilities in these two settings. Interviews would also indicate the feasibility of conducting a survey on health promotion issues in the two settings and to what extent the same questions would be relevant.

Contacting older people living in the community for in-depth interview could be achieved in several ways. Recruiting agencies are able to locate a suitable number of individuals willing to participate, providing the researcher with a sample which reflects the target population. Alternatively, GPs, social services departments or local Age Concern groups may be willing to mail a letter from the researcher to older people on their lists, requesting their participation in the research. For older people living in sheltered housing or retirement housing, wardens may cooperate in a similar way. Whichever method is used, researchers must be able to assure respondents' of the confidentiality of the interviews and anonymity in any report of the research. Screening the initial sample may be necessary to provide the required numbers of people with various illnesses and levels of disability, as well as ensuring a suitable sample in other respects.

For interviews with confused older people, the assistance of a close relative would be required in order to obtain informed consent as far as this is possible. Interviewing a confused older person presents the researcher with a challenge; yet this must be met if the circumstances and feelings of individuals with dementia are not to be neglected (Hunter, 1997). Such interviews can be 'a source of valuable information that may help us better understand the nature of confusion in later life' (McIsaac, 1995: p.4). From the point of view of health promotion, it would be useful to know how coping skills on the part of the older person and their carer(s) can mitigate the effects of memory impairment and improve the quality of life. For the researcher, there is little practical advice on how to proceed with an interview. McIsaac (1995) offers some suggestions which may be helpful and research indicates that the abilities of those labelled as 'confused' are often underestimated (Ripich and Terrell, 1988). Research interest in the nature and management of dementia and in how to communicate with dementing individuals has increased in recent years (for example, see Hoffman and Kaplan *et al.*, 1996; Bell and Troxel, 1997; Tappen, 1997; Hunter, 1997; Harding and Palfrey, 1997). Health promotion research which develops methods of interviewing dementia sufferers would contribute to this growing body of knowledge. However, where dementia is severe, it will be more appropriate to obtain a proxy interview with a carer. Bury and Holme (1990) describe the considerable difficulties in obtaining a nationally representative sample of people aged over 90 for an interview. They note the need for proxy and carer-assisted interviews with demented respondents and the difficulties in communicating with deaf and slightly confused people. Nevertheless they conclude that such research can provide reliable information.

Topics to be explored in in-depth interviews with older people living in the community could include their understanding of the meaning of health; what is most important to their quality of life; how satisfied they are with their situation; feelings about treatment to extend life, compared with palliative care; attitudes to information and recommendations as to healthy behaviour; reasons for health-relevant changes in behaviour; obstacles to such changes; degree of fatalism towards ill health; beliefs about ageing, illness and death; what is seen as most important to their quality of life; what helps them to cope with impairments, practically and psychologically; how well health needs have been met by local agencies, including GP and other health services, social services; and what other aspects of the local environment contribute or otherwise to their wellbeing. Collecting information on respondents' life experience and current circumstances in terms of health status, functional disabilities, material resources, living arrangements, close relationships and informal carers would also be necessary.

Obtaining a suitable sample of older people to interview in a residential setting would require an initial approach to proprietors/ managers of residential and nursing homes. A probability sample of homes could be drawn from lists of registered homes held by selected local authorities and health authorities, with a target of perhaps four residential and two nursing homes where staff and residents agree to participate. A sample of ten residents in each home could be drawn from the list of residents, for in-depth interview. Some consideration of how to minimise perceived differences between researcher and residents is helpful (Fairhurst, 1990). For example, employing older women with appropriate skills to carry out the interviews may improve rapport with residents. The topic areas addressed with older people in the community would need to be modified to reflect the different situation of those living in residential settings.

Interviews with managers and care staff of residential and nursing homes could also be carried out, sampling homes as before but with a larger target number, perhaps 20 homes with three interviews in each. These interviews would provide information on current practice and the perspective of staff in relation to health promotion among residents, including diet, smoking, opportunities for exercise, educational and recreational activities, involvement of residents with the local community and the extent to which residents are encouraged to participate in the running of the home. The interviews would indicate the potential for developing health promotion and how staff perceive the barriers to such programmes. In homes where interviews with both residents and staff were conducted, comparison of views from the two perspectives would be possible, enabling triangulation on issues of health promotion.

Individual in-depth interviews are extremely time-consuming and therefore costly. Although they are essential for some older people, such as those who are particularly frail or confused, focus groups can often be used instead, with gains in the cost-effectiveness of the research.

Focus groups

Focus groups have been widely used in market research but only recently in sociological research. Their value, purpose and method are considered in Morgan (1988; 1993) and Krueger (1994). Although focus groups have been criticised as unrepresentative of the population they are intended to represent, careful recruitment of group participants can provide a sufficiently varied group of people to ensure a wide range of views is encompassed by the research.

Older people may be recruited to focus groups in the same way as for the individual interviews, although a small incentive payment is generally paid to repondents for attendance, as well as travel expenses. It is usually helpful to assemble people of similar age and background into separate groups and to ensure that each meeting place chosen is one in which respondents can feel comfortable as well as being accessible to those who are disabled. Depending on the purpose of the research, groups may be organised on the basis of similar disabilities, or designed to mix people with differing health and functional abilities.

In focus groups, a facilitator guides a discussion among a small group, usually eight to ten people. We would suggest 8–12 focus groups in different parts of the country with older people from various population sub-groups. The facilitator's role is vital in ensuring that the atmosphere is friendly, all members of the group are involved and the discussion remains relevant. Her sensitivity in handling the group is crucial to the success of the event in terms of both the research objectives and the wellbeing of respondents. Discussions with older people with disabilities require careful preparation. For those with impaired hearing, visual materials can supplement verbal communication. For example a flip chart listing the topics to be covered and summarising the views expressed by others in the group can be helpful, while photographs and attitude statements can be used to elicit responses. Care must be taken to ensure that those who are partially sighted are able to join in discussion. An additional assistant is valuable for this and for noting body language to complement the tape recording. Discussions generally last from one-and-a-half to two hours but may need to be shorter for older people.

Similar topics could be included as for the individual interviews, adapted where necessary to the composition of the group. The method shares many of the objectives and advantages of in-depth interviews but differs in offering more insight into the dynamics of opinion-forming and expression. This could be a drawback in that the views of dominant individuals may override or mask those of the more timid. In particular, a fear of expressing attitudes which might be unpopular or of revealing ignorance may inhibit or distort responses in the presence of a group. On the other hand, a group can stimulate the flow of ideas, reveal reactions to disagreement and establish a level of consensus. Moreover, the sharing of experiences in a group can build confidence to express feelings which may have been suppressed in an individual interview (Fielding, 1993).

A major practical advantage of group discussions, as noted above, is that they are considerably cheaper and quicker to conduct than one-to-one interviews with the same number of respondents. Care is needed to obtain a clear recording, using two or more external microphones, to ensure disabled access and to minimise non-attendance. Elderly and disabled people have been found to be particularly likely to fail to attend a group session (Fielding, 1993), although attendance may be improved by providing door-to-door transport.

Summary

Qualitative methods are valuable in researching the health needs of older people in two ways: first, to identify the health issues most salient to older people themselves and to discover their attitudes to changing their lifestyle for health reasons; and second, to inform the construction of suitable questions for a quantitative survey.

Focus groups tend to be more cost-effective than individual in-depth interviews, although they may be difficult to conduct where older people have disabilities which restrict their attendance or participation.

Chapter 7

DESIGNING A QUANTITATIVE SURVEY ON HEALTH PROMOTION ISSUES RELATED TO OLDER PEOPLE

This chapter discusses alternative sample designs and methodological issues which need to be addressed if the HEA wish to commission a survey of the health promotion needs of older people. Previous chapters have illustrated the current state of knowledge about the health and health behaviour of older people, and shown the lack of systematic research on the reasons why older people engage in health promotion activities. Therefore, a quantitative survey should be designed to provide a comprehensive understanding of the factors which encourage and enable older people to engage in health-promoting behaviour and to identify the barriers to a healthy lifestyle. The survey would analyse the variations among older people in their health-related behaviour according to socioeconomic circumstances, gender, marital status and age.

The survey should build on findings from the qualitative work outlined in Chapter 6 and should be informed by findings from the secondary analysis of existing datasets discussed in Chapter 5. Much health-related behaviour is influenced by the social context in which an older person lives. Other members of the household, usually a spouse, may be responsible for food purchase and preparation and their attitudes and behaviour may influence the lifestyle of the older person. It is therefore essential to interview other members of the household as well as the older person.

Age threshold for survey of older people

A key decision will be to determine the appropriate age cut-off point for a quantitative survey of older people. There are a number of alternatives:

(i) Age 50+

This lower age threshold was used by Laslett (1989) and by the influential Carnegie Inquiry into the Third Age (Carnegie Inquiry, 1993). One advantage of using 50 as a minimum age is that many of the practices relevant to health in later life are evident in the fifties. Establishing healthier lifestyles among those in their fifties maximises the potential for improving health later in life.

Another advantage of including those in their fifties is the opportunity to examine the relationships between labour market exit, health, and lifestyle factors. In Britain, men and women increasingly leave the labour market in their fifties. Such 'early exit', although ostensibly due to early retirement, disability or unemployment, is often related to ill health (Kohli *et al.*, 1991; Laczko and Phillipson, 1991). Does early exit from paid employment promote good health, or does it have the reverse effect? And how is the relationship between health and employment status influenced by the social and economic resources at the disposal of men and women in their fifties and early sixties (Ginn and Arber, 1995)? In the USA, the Health and Retirement Survey (HRS) is being undertaken to investigate these issues. It was established in 1992 as a nationally representative sample of 12,600 men and women aged between 51 and 61 (Burkhauser and Gertler, 1995). This government-funded panel survey re-interviews each sample member every two years, in order to analyse the dynamic relationship between health and retirement.

(ii) Age 65+

The conventional definition of older people is age 65, the state pension age for men. Special sections of questions were asked of people aged 65 and over in the General Household Survey in 1980, 1985, 1991 and 1994 (Bennett *et al.*, 1996), which have been the subject of extensive secondary analysis (for example Arber and Ginn, 1990; 1995b). The advantage of restricting a survey to those aged 65 and over, rather than using the threshold of age 50, is that a larger sample of people in the older age groups would be obtained for the same costs. In a representative sample of people aged 50 and over, approximately half will be aged 50–64 and half will be aged 65 and over, see later discussion and Table 7.1.

As the expectation of life increases (see Table 2.1), the majority of people in their late sixties and early seventies will be in good health. It is particularly important to examine in detail the factors influencing the health-related behaviour of these age groups. The more healthy years of later life, prior to the onset of disability and serious illness, are a critical time for promoting health and reducing premature mortality. These ages are also a time when there are very marked social class variations in health (Arber and Ginn, 1993) and in health-promoting behaviour (see Chapter 3); therefore there is considerable room for improving health behaviour among these age groups.

(iii) Age 70+

A quantitative survey restricted to people aged 70 and over would include a high proportion of older people who were already experiencing restrictions of living because of ill health. Such an age threshold would be appropriate if the focus were on promoting health and well-being among older people with some level of disability or chronic illness. Some of the surveys of health behaviour and knowledge have excluded people aged 75 and over, such as the Health Education and Monitoring Survey and the Health and Lifestyle Survey of the UK population discussed in Chapter 5. Future survey research should therefore be designed to collect data on a sufficiently large number of people aged over 70 to allow detailed analysis of variations in their health behaviour, redressing the previous neglect of this important age group. It is imperative to survey these age groups because of the considerable potential for improvement in health and the quality of life at these ages.

In the USA, the Aging and Health in America (AHEAD) study, which started in 1993, is a nationally representative sample of over 8000 people aged 70 and over. The sample is re-interviewed every two years, enabling understanding of the dynamics surrounding increasing disability, economic status (assets and income), the need for and provision of care, family structure and health-related residential and institutional moves. Serious consideration should be given to investing in such large-scale longitudinal studies of ageing and health in Britain (see Chapter 8).

Survey populations

Two possible survey populations are outlined with a recommendation that the HEA should initially focus on the first. These are:

Survey of Older People Living in Private Households
We recommend a nationally representative sample survey of older people aged 50+ (65+ or 70+) living in private households. Such a sample would include people living in sheltered housing, but exclude people living in residential settings. Those living in residential settings are most likely to be in poor health and to suffer from some form of disability so that a survey based on older people in private households will under-estimate the extent of poor health in the total older population. This under-representation becomes increasingly problematic where a survey contains a high proportion of the oldest age groups.

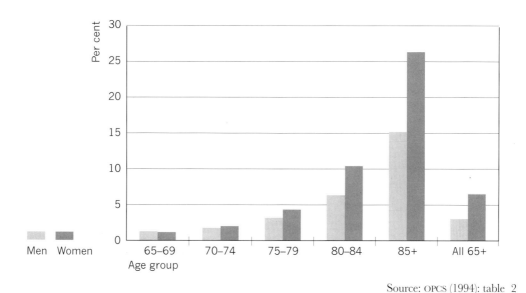

Source: OPCS (1994): table 2

Fig. 7.1. Percentage of men and women in communal establishments – 1991

Survey of Older People Living in Residential Settings

A subsequent survey should be undertaken of a representative sample
of older people (aged 65+ or aged 70+) living in residential settings. A
survey of the health promotion needs of older people in residential settings should focus on the opportunities for undertaking health-
promoting activities relating to lifestyle, exercise, diet and activities
which enhance quality of life, as discussed in Chapter 6.

The likelihood of living in a residential establishment increases
rapidly with advancing age (Arber and Ginn, in press), see Figure 7.1.
Despite the expansion of private residential homes during the 1980s
(Higgs and Victor, 1993), the 1991 population census showed that only
3 per cent of men and 6.4 per cent of women over 65 lived in communal establishments (OPCS, 1993), an increase from 2.5 per cent of
men and 4.6 per cent of women in 1981 (Arber and Ginn, 1991). The
gender differential in communal residence is greater above age 80, and
is particularly pronounced over age 85, when 26 per cent of women
and 15 per cent of men are residents; see Figure 7.1.

An older person's marital status has a very substantial effect on their
likelihood of living in a residential setting; see Figure 7.2. The greater
proportion of older women than men living in residential settings primarily reflects their higher likelihood of being widowed (see Table
2.2b), and not having a partner to care for them should they become
disabled. Residential care is most likely for never married men and
least likely for married men and women, in each age group. For example, in the 65–69 age group, only 0.2 per cent of married people live in

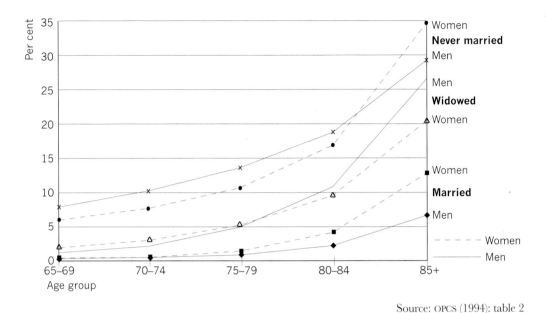

Source: OPCS (1994): table 2

Fig. 7.2. Percentages of older men and women resident in communal establishments in 1991 by marital status and age groups

a communal establishment compared with 8 per cent of single men and 6 per cent of single women. Even among those over 85, four times more single men (29 per cent) than married men (7 per cent) live in a residential setting, as do three times more single women (35 per cent) than married women (13 per cent). The widowed are in an intermediate position in each age group. These differences reflect the selective entry into residential care of older people on the basis of both ill health and marital status. Marital status is a predictor of the availability of informal carers, including both having a spouse and children, to support the older person.

A survey of older people in residential care will disproportionately contain women, and older people who are never married, widowed and divorced, whereas a survey of older people living in private households will omit those older people in the poorest health, because of their selection into residential establishments. This selectivity on health grounds is less for married older people, who on average are more likely to remain living at home despite high levels of disability (Figure 7.2).

It is recommended that a survey of older people in residential settings should be undertaken at a later stage in this HEA programme of research, following a quantitative survey of older people in private households. Therefore, this review will not discuss the sampling strategy for a survey of older people living in residential settings.

Sampling strategy for survey of older people living in the community

The proposed survey of older people living in the community would include people aged 50 and over (or 70 and over) living in private households, including older people living in sheltered (and warden-assisted) housing. Probability sampling is recommended rather than quota sampling. Use of quota controls often fails to ensure a representative sample of older people, inadequately representing older age groups. The recommended sampling frame for sample selection is the Postcode Address File, which provides a more up-to-date coverage of all addresses than the Electoral Register (Lynn and Lievesley, 1991).

An alternative method would be to use general practitioners' age-sex registers as a sampling frame. This would be of greater value for a sample of people aged 70 and above than for a sample of people aged 50 and over, because of the higher costs of operating an age-eligibility screen (as discussed below) when the proportion of addresses containing age-eligible individuals is lower. If general practitioners' age-sex registers were used, it would be necessary to select a widely dispersed sample of general practices, both geographically and in terms of the socioeconomic characteristics of areas. Ideally, it would be desirable to sample from at least 50 practices. To do so would entail costs of approaching 50 practices and negotiating access to their lists, and possibly obtaining ethical committee approval as well. General practitioners are usually reluctant to give researchers lists of the names and addresses of patients and may insist that they make the initial contact. If such a strategy was required, this would probably lower the overall response rate, and make the final sample less representative.

The appropriate sample size will depend on the amount of statistical power needed for various types of analyses of specific sub-groups within the sample, as well as the available budget for the survey. Our recommendation is that the minimum usable survey size would be 3000 people aged 50 and over or 1500 people aged 70 and over.

The remainder of this section assumes that the Postcode Address File will be used as a sampling frame. Table 7.1a illustrates that a probability sample of 4000 people aged 50 and over living in private households would result in half the sample being aged 50–64 and half over age 65. Since it is particularly important in the proposed study to include a sufficiently large number of people aged over 70, we recommend that people over age 65 are oversampled by a factor of two. This disproportionate sample selection would mean that approximately 1000 people in the sample were aged 50–64 and 2000 aged over 65,

Table 7.1a. Characteristics of a representative sample of 4000 people aged 50 and over living in private households

Age range	Numbers			Percentages		
	Men	Women	All	Men	Women	All
50–64	970	1010	1980	24.3	25.2	49.5
65–74	540	660	1200	13.5	16.5	30.0
75+	300	520	820	7.5	15.5	20.5
Total	1810	2190	4000	42.3	54.7	100%

Estimates based on sample obtained from the General Household Survey for 1992–94.

Table 7.1b. Characteristics of a disproportionate stratified sample of 3010 people aged 50 and over living in private households

Age range	Numbers			Percentages		
	Men	Women	All	Men	Women	All
50–64	485	505	990	16.1	16.8	32.9
65–74	540	660	1200	17.9	21.9	39.9
75+	300	520	820	10.0	17.3	27.2
Total	1325	1685	3010	44.0	56.0	100%

Note. Assuming people aged 50–64 have half the chance of selection compared to people aged 65 and over.

Estimates based on sample obtained from the General Household Survey for 1992–94.

Table 7.2. Characteristics of a representative sample of 3000 people aged 70 and over living in private households

Age range	Numbers			Percentages		
	Men	Women	All	Men	Women	All
70–74	555	705	1260	18.5	23.5	42.0
75–79	321	474	795	10.7	15.8	26.5
80–84	222	363	585	7.4	12.1	19.5
85+	102	258	360	3.4	8.6	12.0
Total	1000	2000	3000	40.0	60.0	100%

Estimates based on sample obtained from the General Household Survey for 1992–94.

reducing the total sample size from 4000 to about 3000 (see Table 7.1b). This would reduce the cost of the survey substantially while having little adverse effect on the precision of estimates of the health behaviour of different age groups among the older population.

If a survey population of 3000 older people aged 70 and over were required, Table 7.2 shows the estimated number and proportion of people in each age and sex category. Sixty per cent of the sample would be women and 40 per cent men. There is a declining number and proportion of people in each five-year age group; for example, the numbers vary from 1260 aged 70–74 to 360 aged 85 and over. Also, the gender balance becomes more weighted towards women as age increases.

Sample selection

We recommend that the sample is drawn using Probability Proportional to Size (PPS) sampling based on postal sectors, previously stratified according to region, the age structure and socioeconomic characteristics of the postal sector (Lynn and Lievesley, 1991). Postcodes and addresses would then be selected from within the sampled postal sectors using the Postcode Address File. At selected addresses it would be necessary to use a short screening questionnaire to determine if anyone at that address fulfilled the age criteria of eligibility for inclusion in the sample.

At each selected address, all persons within the specified age range would be interviewed. In addition, we would recommend interviewing spouses who were younger than the specified age criteria. For example, this practice was used in the DSS Retirement and Retirement Plans Survey which interviewed all persons aged 55–69 living at a representative sample of addresses, and also interviewed their partners who were outside this age range (Bone *et al.*, 1992). This procedure would result in an achieved sample somewhat higher than 3000.

In order to achieve a sample size of 3000 aged 50 and over (or aged 70 and over), it would be necessary to estimate the age-eligibility rate within sample addresses. This would be approximately 35 per cent for people aged 50 and over, and approximately 14 per cent for people aged 70 and over. Thus, the cost of age screening would be higher for a sample of people aged 70 and over than for a sample of people aged 50 and over, because more sample addresses contain someone over 50 than someone over 70.

The study would interview all people aged above the age threshold in sample addresses. For people aged 50–64, about 80 per cent are married or live with another adult, whereas for people aged 75–84 under half are married or live with another adult, and at age 85 and over, 60 per cent live alone. This variation in marital status by age means that two interviews with older people are more likely in households containing people aged 50–64 than in households containing people aged 80 and over. For example, a sample of 1000 people aged

50–64 would be found in about 550 households, but a sample of 1000 people aged 70 and over would be drawn from a sample of over 700 households.

To determine the required number of addresses to select from the Postcode Address File it would be necessary to estimate the age-eligibility rate at sampled addresses, the expected response rate (probably around 75 per cent) and the expected average number of eligible respondents at each selected address. The latter would be greater for younger than for older age groups.

Development of the interview schedule

The survey interview schedule would be developed following qualitative research, as outlined in Chapter 6. The interview schedule would be structured in sections on a range of topics relating to health, disability, health-related behaviour, attitudes, barriers to health-promoting behaviour, socioeconomic resources, and aspects of the quality of the local environment in relation to health behaviour. The survey would seek explanations for older people's health-related behaviour and identify how obstacles to health-promoting behaviour may be overcome.

The survey questions will build on existing questionnaires, such as questions used in the Health and Lifestyle Surveys, the Health Education and Monitoring Survey and the Health Survey for England, but will also include a series of questions which probe the reasons for health-related behaviours. The questionnaire will be largely precoded, but will also contain open questions which are field coded by the interviewer. A pilot study of approximately 100 interviews should be undertaken.

Interviewing

A high response rate is essential if this research is to have a major impact on policy relating to the health of older people. The response rate may be maximised if older people act as interviewers (aged 50–65), since they have been found to have better rapport with older people (Fisk and Abbott, 1997). The subject matter of the research is likely to be of considerable interest to older people, since health is one of their major concerns (Bearon, 1989), and respondents are likely to see the research as having beneficial consequences. A high response rate of at least 75 per cent is likely, even though older people have been found to have a lower response rate in market research (Burton, 1996). This lower response is mainly because older people are less interested in being involved in market research studies and see such studies as of less relevance to themselves than is the case for younger age groups (Windle and Mouncey, 1997).

Research has shown that pre-notification, whereby the respondent is sent a letter about the survey in advance of the interviewer's contact, increases the response rate (Windle and Mouncey, 1997). Letters in advance tend to legitimise the survey by reducing suspicion, and should be used in this research. It will be essential for interviewers to display identification to respondents to allay any suspicions by older people that the interviewers may not be bona fide.

The training of interviewers is crucial for obtaining a high response rate and good quality data from older people. It will be essential to train interviewers in how to approach older people, to be perceptive about whether the older person has physical or mental conditions which may affect their ability to understand and respond, as discussed in Chapter 6. Interviewers must be sensitive to ethical issues surrounding research with older people (Peace, 1990).

If an older person is too ill or mentally frail to be interviewed, interviewers will be instructed to perform a partial interview which only contains key questions. In circumstances where this is not feasible or acceptable to the older person, a proxy interview should be obtained with another household member, or with the person who is primarily responsible for providing care or support to the older person. Proxy interviews will contain a reduced number of questions, primarily factual questions about the older person's health, disability status, socio-economic circumstances and health behaviour. They will not contain attitudinal questions, which cannot be asked on behalf of another person. For research with older people, it is essential to specify procedures for the use of proxy interviews to ensure that older people who are ill or mentally frail are not under-represented in the survey.

Summary

Two alternative nationally representative quantitative surveys are proposed: 1. a survey of 3000 people aged over 50, which would include over-sampling of people aged 65 and over, and 2. a sample of 3000 people aged 70 and over. For both surveys, a probability sample is recommended based on selection of a national sample of addresses from the Postcode Address File. A short screening interview would be used to identify addresses containing age-eligible respondents. Interviewers would need to be trained to be aware of the special issues associated with interviewing mentally or physically frail older people.

Chapter 8

THE NEED FOR A PANEL OR LONGITUDINAL SURVEY OF OLDER PEOPLE'S HEALTH

Cross-sectional data on older people's health and mortality have established the prevalence of various types of ill health according to class, ethnicity, gender, region and local area but leave important questions unanswered as to causal processes.

The first of these concerns the compression of morbidity thesis (Fries, 1980; 1989) that better health in successive cohorts will lead to delayed onset and shorter duration of morbidity (see Chapter 2). Cross-sectional surveys can show whether the prevalence of illness of various kinds is increasing or decreasing for given age groups but longitudinal data are needed to measure the duration of ill health and to separate cohort from age effects. Minimising morbidity is important both in reducing the distress of older individuals and in its implications for the projection of future costs of health and social care. It is remarkable that there has been so little attempt in Britain to answer this question, given the spate of rhetoric and alarmist panic about the growth in the older population. This contrasts with the USA, where the longitudinal surveys of Health and Retirement (HRS) and Aging and Health (AHEAD) were started in the early 1990s (Burkhauser and Gertler, 1995); see Chapter 7.

Second, the reasons for structured variations in health expectancy are uncertain because of a lack of information on the sequencing of events and health conditions. Higher social class is associated with better health and with a healthier lifestyle but how are these causally related? Opportunities for healthy living are socially structured. For example, a certain level of income is needed for the middle-class norm of a healthy diet, adequate heating, living in a pollution-free residential area and participation in social activities, sports, health clubs and adult education. Moreover, those from manual occupations are more likely to be exposed to stresses and hazards during their working life which contribute to ill health in later life and constrain attempts to maintain levels of physical exercise.

A longitudinal survey, in which the same questions were asked of a panel of older people after an interval, could trace the process of health change in older people over time, illuminating such questions as how changes in lifestyle affect health, how the onset of frailty or bereavement influence activities, relationships and living arrangements, and to what extent people recover from disabling conditions.

In this chapter, we examine the potential of existing British surveys with a longitudinal element. These include the British Household Panel Survey, the Health and Lifestyle Survey and the Retirement and Retirement Plans Survey. The Health Survey for England, although currently an annual cross-sectional survey, could potentially be adapted to follow up a panel of older people.

British Household Panel Survey, annual since 1991

The British Household Panel Survey (BHPS) provides a unique source of longitudinal information that can be used to examine aspects of change in people's lives, including a limited range of questions on health. Data are collected about individual and household characteristics, with a focus placed on the significant factors affecting change at a micro-social level.

The original panel sample in 1991 included individuals from approximately 5000 households (and 10,000 individual interviews) in Great Britain (Taylor, 1992; Buck *et al.*, 1994); see Chapter 5. These same individuals are re-interviewed annually in successive waves. The design of the BHPS allows for changes in household composition over time. If an individual leaves the household then they are followed to their new home. Similarly, new additions to the household are added to the sample along with children when they reach the age of 16 years. The data are re-weighted to adjust for a differential non-response amongst original panel members, thus ensuring that the panel retains the characteristics of a nationally representative sample.

All waves of the data from 1991 to 1997 could be used to capture the dynamic aspects of health and socioeconomic status that cannot be estimated using cross-sectional data. The panel design also incorporates retrospective information on changes in life circumstances in the preceding year. For each wave of the survey, the proportion of the sample aged over 65 years (nearly 1800 at wave 1) remains consistently above 20 per cent and the size of this age group has increased by 4.5 per cent between wave 1 and wave 5. Although the oldest members of the panel have died since the start of the survey, nearly one-quarter of older people interviewed in 1991 were re-interviewed in wave 5.

Health and Caring are main topic areas covered by the BHPS but research use of these data has been notably lacking, even though the design of the health record relates to some of the key issues in the Health of the Nation report (Department of Health, 1992). Data are collected on morbidity, the use of primary health care and aspects of health behaviour. Also included is the 12-item General Health Questionnaire which examines psychological wellbeing. Relating this health information to the older population, the BHPS can be used to investigate how life events, such as widowhood or retirement, affect mental and physical wellbeing. In addition, changes in health status can be related to changes in social and economic circumstances such as the financial position of the individual or household. Examining these changes over a six-year period would highlight any time-lag effects between changing life circumstances and health status.

Health and Lifestyles Survey, 1984/5 and 1991/2

The original Health and Lifestyle Survey conducted in 1984/5 (HALS1) is described in Chapter 5. The follow-up survey in 1991/2 (HALS2) was carried out in order to realise the potential of a longitudinal study in revealing relationships between lifestyles and health.

Whereas HALS1 only covered those living in their own homes, thus excluding the more frail individuals, all survivors among the original sample were eligible for inclusion in HALS2, even if they were in hospital or living in a residential or nursing home. Attrition reduced the original sample of 9003 (HALS1) to 5352 (HALS2). Because HALS1 is 'flagged' with the National Health Service Register, the dates and causes of deaths of respondents can be added to the dataset. The follow-up survey repeated all the questions and measurements made in the first survey, adding new questions about the respondent's experience of change over the previous seven years.

The two waves of HALS allow analysis of changes in health, health knowledge and health behaviour, relating these to material and social circumstances. The editors note that, 'some attempt can also be made to identify the effect of change in individual circumstances upon physical and mental health' (Cox, Huppert and Whichelow, 1993: p.x). However, the number of older people in the panel is rather small for such analyses, just over 1000 aged 60 or over in 1984/5. The gap of seven years is too long to capture some changes and the 1991/2 survey is now six years old and becoming increasingly out of date.

Retirement and Retirement Plans, 1988 and 1994

The Retirement and Retirement Plans Survey (RRP) provides a means of tracing the development of disability in the older population. The first survey, in 1988/9, interviewed a sample of over 3500 men and women aged 55–69 living in private households in Great Britain, and also interviewed about 600 partners outside this age range (Bone *et al.*, 1992). This panel was surveyed again in 1994 (Goldman, 1994), providing longitudinal data over a six-year period on disability, as well as changes in current income, economic activity, occupational class, educational qualifications and household characteristics. The second wave comprised interviews with over 2200 surviving respondents aged 61–76. A fifth of respondents were widowed between the two interviews.

Both waves include a detailed section on the informant's disability status. This was based on questions in the OPCS surveys of disability (Martin, Meltzer and Elliot, 1988), which identified thirteen areas of possible disability: locomotion, reaching and stretching, dexterity, personal care, continence, hearing, seeing, communication, behaviour, intellectual functioning, consciousness, eating and disfigurement. The inclusion of questions on mental functions adds an important dimension to the measurement of disability, in terms of the implications for social care. A single score measuring the severity of disability was developed, based on the severity in the individual's three highest scoring areas of disability. In addition, information on timing of exit from the labour force and on detailed employment histories is available, enabling disability to be related to past and current employment.

For married people, information on disability is collected from both partners, allowing identification of couples where both partners are disabled, with implications for their capacity to provide adequate informal care for each other.

A major advantage of the RRP's longitudinal data is that information is available as to the age of onset of disability for all individuals, as well as on their level of disability at each interview. It will be possible to trace the process of becoming disabled and to measure the loss of functional abilities over time and the extent to which individuals recover partially or fully from their disability.

Health Survey for England, 1991 onwards

The Health Survey for England (HSE), an annual survey of adults aged 16 and over living in private households in Britain, is described in detail in Chapter 5 and some of the findings concerning older people are examined in Chapter 3. As an alternative to funding a wholly new longitudinal survey on older people's health, a longitudinal element could be added by following up all older people first interviewed in 1995 (or another year) at intervals, as was done with the Health and Lifestyle Survey (Cox, Huppert and Whichelow, 1993).

A longitudinal extension of the HSE would provide relevant information on the issues identified in the introduction to this chapter. From 1993, it provides extensive information on over 5500 individuals aged over 55 (3200 over 65), relating to diet, exercise, body mass, smoking and drinking, as well as psycho-social health and social support. Physiological measures include blood tests for cholesterol, anaemia and fibrinogen. The emphasis of the HSE for 1991–4 is somewhat different from 1995–6, the focus shifting from cardiovascular disease to respiratory conditions. If a panel were followed up it would clearly be desirable to use as baseline a year in which a comprehensive core of questions on health and health behaviour is asked.

Summary

Each of the three existing longitudinal datasets has potential for secondary analysis to reveal the relationships between changes in circumstances, health and health behaviour of older people. However, each has some drawbacks: the British Household Panel Survey, although providing information on self-assessed health for 1800 people over 65, has little information about functional disability. The Retirement and Retirement Plans Survey has a good range of health questions and includes 2200 people over 61 but the maximum age of 76 in 1994 limits its usefulness in understanding advanced old age.

The Health and Lifestyle Survey (HALS), although its questions and measures are comprehensive, has a rather small number of respondents, only 1000 aged over 60, and relates to the situation some time ago. The annual Health Survey for England provides excellent information on all aspects of health and health behaviour and includes 3200 individuals aged over 65. If extended by following up older people at one- or two-yearly intervals it would provide a most valuable longitudinal dataset in the future.

Chapter 9

RECOMMENDATIONS AND CONCLUSIONS

Older people's health is becoming a matter of key policy interest, fuelled by increasing longevity and a concern that this is matched by increased years of healthy life. However, older people have been largely neglected in terms of health promotion. This review outlines the current state of knowledge about older people's health and health behaviour and provides recommendations for future research to redress this imbalance.

There is a lack of detailed research evidence about the health-related behaviour of older people, in terms of their lifestyles, smoking, drinking, diet and exercise. Nor is it clear to what extent the factors associated with a healthy lifestyle among the older population are similar to those among younger age groups and what older people perceive as the barriers to a healthy lifestyle.

Before concerted action to promote older people's health can be effectively introduced it is necessary to undertake further baseline research to identify the health promotion needs of older people, and the ways in which social, economic and environmental factors impinge on their attitudes and opportunities for engaging in health-promoting behaviour. In this way it will be feasible to design effective health promotion strategies.

Recommendations

To answer the pressing questions about the health needs and health promotion issues relating to older people, it is recommended that the Health Education Authority adopt a programme of research involving a three-stage strategy.

Stage 1: Secondary analysis of existing datasets

The potential of secondary analysis and the strengths and weaknesses of a range of datasets were outlined in Chapter 5. During 1997–8, secondary analysis of national datasets should be conducted to identify the target groups of older people with particularly poor health and those who are most likely to be engaging in health-damaging behaviour.

The three most important national data sources for secondary analysis are:

1. The Health Survey for England, 1993, 1994 and 1995, which can be analysed to provide detailed data on the health status and health

risk factors (smoking, drinking, diet, obesity and exercise) of five-year age groups of older people and how these vary with their socio-economic characteristics, marital status and living arrangements;

2. The General Household Survey for 1993, 1994 and 1995 can provide detailed information on the health status of older people, their use of primary and secondary care services and their smoking and drinking (in 1994). In addition, in 1994, people aged 65+ were asked a special section of questions, focusing on their level of disability and receipt of community health and welfare services;

3. The Health Education and Monitoring Survey 1995 allows analysis of the health attitudes and beliefs about disease prevention and their own health status among people aged 55–74. This will show whether the underlying beliefs about health-promoting or health-damaging behaviour differ among people aged 65–74, people aged 55–64 and younger age groups. The socioeconomic correlates of health attitudes can be analysed, contrasting older and younger age groups.

Stage 2: Qualitative research

The value of qualitative research was discussed in Chapter 6. A high priority for 1997–98 will be to conduct a series of focus groups with older people to elucidate the factors associated with involvement in health-damaging behaviour and the constraints they face in seeking to change their behaviour. Focus groups should probe both health behaviour which is under the individual's control and also wider social and environmental factors which may damage their health and quality of life or prevent them from engaging in health-promoting behaviour, for example the safety of their neighbourhood, quality of the local environment and the ways in which limited financial resources influence opportunities for behavioural change.

Focus groups provide older people with the opportunity to raise issues of relevance to themselves and to define the barriers to promoting their better health. Analysis of data from these focus groups is a necessary stage for designing a clearly targeted interview survey of the health needs and health promotion issues relevant to older people.

Stage 3: A national survey of older people's health needs and health promotion issues

The proposed methodology for a large-scale national survey of older people's health needs and health promotion issues was outlined in Chapter 7. Such a survey should build on the secondary analysis and qualitative work undertaken during 1997–98. The survey should be designed and piloted during late 1998 and fielded in early 1999.

The target age group and number of survey interviews will depend on the scale of available funding. Ideally the survey should cover all people aged 50 and over, with a double sampling fraction for people aged 65 and over (see Chapter 7), but available resources may make a survey of people aged over 70 the most cost-effective strategy for the HEA to adopt. The topics to be covered in such a survey should be finalised following the results of the secondary analysis and qualitative phases of the programme of research.

Conclusions

To date in Britain, health promotion among older people has been largely neglected by health educators and policymakers. Promoting older people's health requires an awareness of the factors influencing older people's lifestyle as well as recognition of the impact of structural influences on their health. A danger is that too great an emphasis on health promotion centred on individual behavioural change may lead to older people being blamed for their ill health. It is important to recognise that many of the causes of ill health are outside the individual's control, including material circumstances and the nature of the local environment.

Extensive research evidence shows that older people's health differs according to their occupational class, current material circumstances, gender, ethnicity and area of residence. Despite the fact that there are wide variations in health among five-year age groups in the older population, age alone is an inadequate predictor of health – other socioeconomic factors are equally important. It is essential not to treat older people as a homogeneous group but to recognise and understand this diversity in any approaches to health promotion.

The health of older people can be most effectively promoted through a partnership approach in which health education and other initiatives addressed at individuals are combined with social policies to improve older people's standard of living and access to appropriate health and social care. It is essential that older people's own perspectives are taken into account in policies to promote their health.

APPENDIX

Health-related topics included in existing surveys

This appendix details the main topic areas for each of the main datasets covered in Chapter 5 and where appropriate indicates the year in which the topic was included in the survey.

1. Health Education and Monitoring Survey 1995 (HEMS)

Morbidity: Long-standing illness, limiting long-standing illness, general health.
Utilisation: GP consultations.
Health attitudes and beliefs: Disease prevention, knowledge.
Health behaviour: Smoking, drinking, physical activity, nutrition.
Socioeconomic background: Social class, educational level, housing tenure, car ownership, ethnic origin.

2. Health and Lifestyle Survey 1984/5 and 1991/2 (HALS)

Morbidity: Long-standing illness, limiting long-standing illness, general health, cognitive tests, psycho-social factors, physiological measurements.
Utilisation: Receipt of prescription, treatment of health complaints.
Health attitudes and beliefs: Knowledge about causes and risks of ill health.
Health behaviour: Nutrition, drinking, smoking, exercise, work and leisure.
Socioeconomic background: Accommodation, housing tenure, income, education,* employment,* ethnic origin (coded by interviewer).

3. Health and Lifestyle Survey of the UK population 1992 (MORI)

Morbidity: General health, long-standing illness, limiting long-standing illness, psycho-social health.
Utilisation: GP consultations: access, purpose, problems discussed, satisfaction with service.
Health attitudes and beliefs: Disease prevention.
Health behaviour: Smoking, buying food.
Socioeconomic background: Housing tenure, car ownership, household income, education, employment status,† ethnic origin and background.

* Information collected for individual and spouse/partner
† Information collected from all household members

[78]

4. Health Survey for England 1991–1996 (HSE)

Morbidity: General health, long-standing illness, limiting long-standing illness, psycho-social health (includes GHQ), physiological measurements.

Utilisation: Prescribed medication.

Special topic areas: Cardiovascular disease (1991–94), asthma and related conditions (1995–96), accidents (1995–96), disability (1995).

Health behaviour: Diet and nutrition (1993–94), smoking, drinking, physical activity.

Socioeconomic background: Housing tenure, car availability, educational level, employment status, ethnic origin.

5. General Household Survey (GHS)

Morbidity: Long-standing illness, limiting long-standing illness, general health, acute sickness.

Utilisation: GP consultations, inpatient and outpatient attendances, number of inpatient stays.

Special topic areas: Informal carers (1985 and 1990), persons aged 65+ (1980,1985,1991,1994), accidents (1987–89), mobility aids (1993)

Health behaviour: Smoking and drinking (alternate years).

Socioeconomic background: Housing tenure, accommodation, car ownership, consumer durables, education, employment, income, social class, ethnic origin.

REFERENCES

Abella, R. and Heslin, R. (1984) 'Health, locus of control, values and the behaviour of family and friends: an integrated approach to understanding health behaviour', *Basic and Applied Social Psychology*, **5**: 283–93.

Activity and Health Research (1992) *Allied Dunbar National Fitness Survey: Main Findings*. London: Sports Council and Health Education Authority.

Age Concern (1995) *Hospital Afterthought: Support for Older People discharged from Hospital*. London: Age Concern.

Ageing Well Europe (1996) *A European Programme of Health Promotion for and with Older People*. London: Age Concern.

Allan, G. and Adams, R. (1989) 'Aging and the structure of friendship'. In Adams, R. and Blieszner, R. (eds). *Older Adult Friendship*. London: Sage, pp. 45–64.

Anderson, R. and Bury, M. (eds) (1988) *Living with Chronic Illness: the Experience of Patients and their Families*. London: Unwin Hyman.

Arber, S. (1987) 'Social class, non-employment and chronic illness: continuing the health inequalities debate', *British Medical Journal*, **294**: 1067–73.

Arber, S. (1996) 'Integrating non-employment into research on health inequalities', *International Journal of Health Services*, **26**(3): 445–81.

Arber, S. (1997) 'Comparing inequalities in women's and men's health: Britain in the 1990s', *Social Science and Medicine*, **44**: 773–87.

Arber, S. and Ginn, J. (1990) 'The meaning of informal care: gender and the contribution of older people', *Ageing and Society*, **12**(4): 429–54.

Arber, S. and Ginn, J. (1991) *Gender and Later Life: a Sociological Analysis of Resources and Constraints*. London: Sage.

Arber, S. and Ginn, J. (1993) 'Gender and inequalities in health in later life'. In Stacey, M. and Olensen, V. (eds) *Social Science and Medicine:* Special issue on Women, men and health, **36** (1) 33–46.

Arber, S. and Ginn, J. (1995a) 'Gender differences in the relationship between paid employment and informal care', *Work, Employment and Society*, **9**(3): 445–71.

Arber, S. and Ginn, J. (1995b) 'Gender differences in informal care', *Health and Social Care in the Community*, **3**: 19–31.

Arber, S. and Ginn, J. (in press) 'Health and illness in later life'. In Field, D. and Taylor, S. (eds) *Sociological Perspectives on Health and Illness*. London: Blackwell Scientific.

Askham, J., Henshaw, L. and Tarpey, M. (1993) 'Policies and perceptions of identity: service needs of elderly people from black and ethnic minority backgrounds'. In Arber, S. and Evandrou, M. (eds) *Ageing, Independence and the Life Course*. London: Jessica Kingsley.

Association of Metropolitan Authorities (1994) *A Survey of Social Services Charging Policies 1992–4*. London: AMA.

Association of Metropolitan Authorities and Association of County Councils (1995) *Who Gets Community Care: a Survey of Community Care Eligibility Criteria*. London: AMA/ACC.

Atchley, R. (1980) *The Social Forces in Later Life*. Belmont, Calif.: Wadsworth.

Balarajan, R. and Bulusi, L. (1990) 'Mortality among immigrants in England and Wales, 1979–83'. In Britton, M. (ed.) *Mortality and Geography: a Review in the Mid-1980s*, OPCS Series DS No. 9. London: HMSO, pp. 103–21.

Bankoff, E. (1983) 'Social support and adaptation to widowhood', *Journal of Marriage and the Family*, **45**: 827–39.

Barker, J. (1984) *Black and Asian Old People in Britain*. Mitcham: Age Concern England.

Baylor, A. and Spirdoso, W. (1988) 'Systematic aerobic exercise and components of reaction time in older women', *Journals of Gerontology*, **43**(5): 121–6.

Bearon, L. B. (1989) 'No great expectations: the underpinnings of life satisfaction for older women', *Gerontologist*, **29**(6): 772–84.

Beers, M., Fink, A. and Beck, J. (1991) 'Screening recommendations for the elderly', *American Journal of Public Health*, **81**(9): 1131–40.

Beisecker, A. and Thompson, T. (1995) 'The elderly patient–physician interaction'. Chapter in Nussbaum, J. and Coupland, J. (eds), *Handbook of Communication and Aging Research*. Mahwah, New Jersey: Lawrence Erlbaum.

Bennett, G. and Ebrahim, S. (1992) *The Essentials of Health Care of the Elderly*. London: Edward Arnold.

Bennett, N., Dodd, T., Flatley, J., Freeth, S. and Bolling, K. (1995) *Health Survey for England 1993*. Social Survey Division of OPCS. London: HMSO.

Bennett, N., Jarvis, L., Rowlands, O., Singleton, N. and Haselden, L. (1996) *Living in Britain: Results from the 1994 General Household Survey*, OPCS. London: HMSO.

Berg, R. and Cassells, J. (1990) *The Second Fifty Years: Promoting Health and Preventing Disability*. Washington: National Academy Press.

Berkman, L. and Breslow, L. (1983) *Health and Ways of Living*. Oxford: Oxford University Press.

Berkman, L. and Syme, S. (1979) 'Social networks, host resistance and mortality: a nine year follow up of Alameda County residents', *American Journal of Epidemiology*, **109**: 186–204.

Blakemore, K. (1989) 'Does age matter? The case of old age in minority ethnic groups'. In Bytheway, B., Keil, T., Allatt, P. and Bryman, A. (eds). *Becoming and Being Old: Sociological Approaches to Later Life*. London: Sage, pp. 158–75.

Blakemore, K. and Boneham, M. (1993) *Ageing and Ethnicity*. Buckingham: Open University Press.

Blane, D., Davey Smith, G. and Bartley, M. (1990) 'Social class differences in years of potential life lost: size, trends and principal causes', *British Medical Journal*, **301**: 429–32.

Blaxter, M. (1990) *Health and Lifestyles*. London and New York: Tavistock/ Routledge.

Blazer, D. (1982) 'Social support and mortality in an elderly community population', *American Journal of Epidemiology*, **115**: 684–94.

Blumenthal, J., Emery, C., Madden, D., George, L., Coleman, R., Riddle, M., McKee, D., Reasoner, J. and Williams, R. (1989) 'Cardiovascular and behavioural effects of aerobic exercise training on the health of older men and women', *Journal of Gerontology*, **44**(5): M147–57.

Bone, M., Gregory, J., Gill, B. and Lader, D. (1992) *Retirement and Retirement Plans Survey*, DSS. London: HMSO.

Bone, M., Bebbington, A., Jagger, C., Morgan, K. and Nicolaas, G. (1995) *Health Expectancy and its Uses*. London: HMSO.

Bowling, B. (1990) *Elderly People from Ethnic Minorities: a Report on Four Projects*. London: Age Concern Institute of Gerontology.

Bowling, A. (1995) 'What things are important in people's lives?: a survey of the public's judgements to inform scales of health related quality of life', *Social Science and Medicine*, **41**(10): 1447–62.

Breeze, E., Trevor, G. and Wilmot, A. (eds)(1991) *General Household Survey 1989*, OPCS Series, GHS No. 20. London: HMSO.

Breeze, E., Maidment, A., Bennett, N., Flatley, J. and Carey, S. (1994) *Health Survey for England 1992*. Social Survey Division of OPCS. London: HMSO.

Bridgwood, A., Malbon, G., Lader, D. and Matheson, J. (1996) *Health in England 1995: What People Know, What People Think and What People Do*. London: HEA.

Brown, G. and Harris, T. (1978) *The Social Origins of Depression*. London: Tavistock.

Buck, N., Gershuny, J., Rose, D. and Scott, J. (1994) *Changing Households: the British Household Panel Survey 1990–92*. Colchester: University of Essex ESRC Centre on Microsocial Change.

Burkhauser, R. V. and Gertler, P. J. (1995) 'The Health and Retirement Survey', *Journal of Human Resources*, Special issue: **30**: 1–318.

Burton, J. (1996) *Public Attitudes and Responses to Survey Research: a Review of the Literature*. Market Research Society.

Bury, M. and Holme, A. (1990) 'Researching very old people'. In Peace, S. (ed.) *Researching Social Gerontology: Concepts, Methods and Issues*. London: Sage, chapter 9.

Butler, R. and Lewis, M. (1976) *Love and Sex after 60*. New York: Harper & Row.

Cameron, E., Evers, H., Badger, H. and Atkin, A. (1989) 'Black old women, disability and health carers'. In Jefferys, M. (ed.) *Growing Old in the Twentieth Century*. London: Routledge, pp. 230–48.

Caplan, G. (1974) *Social Support and Community Mental Health*. New York: Basic Books.

Carnegie Inquiry (1993) *Health and Function in the Third Age*, Papers prepared for the Carnegie Inquiry into the Third Age. London: Nuffield Provincial Hospitals Trust.

Carp, F. and Christensen, D. (1986) 'Technical environmental assessment predictors of residential satisfaction: a study of elderly women living alone', *Research on Aging*, **8**(2): 269–87.

Carter, T. and Nash, C. (1992) *Pensioners' Voice: an Active Voice*. Guildford: Pre-Retirement Association.

Cassel, J. (1976) 'The contribution of the social environment to host resistance', *American Journal of Epidemiology*, **104**: 107–23.

Cohen, S. and Syme, L. (eds) (1985) *Social Support and Health*. New York: Academic Press.

Cohen, S. and Willis, T. (1985) 'Stress, social support and the buffering hypothesis', *Psychological Bulletin*, **98**(2): 310–57.

Colhoun, H. and Prescott-Clarke, P. (eds) (1996) *Health Survey for England 1994*. London: HMSO.

Collins, K. (1986) 'Low indoors temperature and morbidity in the elderly', *Age and Aging*, **15**(4): 212–20.

Cox, B. D., Blaxter, M., Buckle, A., Fenner, N., Golding, J., Gore, M., Huppert, F., Nickson, J., Roth, M., Stark, J., Wadsworth, M. and Whichelow, M. (1987) *The Health and Lifestyle Survey*. London: The Health Promotion Research Trust.

Cox, B. (1993a) 'Trends in blood pressure and respiratory function'. In Cox, B., Huppert, F. and Wichelow, M., chapter 5.

Cox, B. (1993b) 'Changes in body measurements'. In Cox, B., Huppert, F. and Wichelow, M., chapter 6.

Cox, B. and Whichelow, M. (1993) 'Changes in exercise and leisure activities'. In Cox, B., Huppert, F. and Wichelow, M., chapter 14.

Cox, B., Huppert, F. and Whichelow, M. (eds) (1993) *The Health and Lifestyle Survey: Seven Years On*. Aldershot: Dartmouth.

Crohan, S. and Antonucci, T. (1989) 'Friends as a source of support in old age'. In Adams, R. and Blieszner, R. (eds), *Older Adult Friendship*. London: Sage, pp. 129–46.

Dale, A., Arber, S., Procter, M. (1988) *Doing Secondary Analysis*. Contemporary Social Research: 17. London: Unwin Hyman.

Dalley, G., Howse, K., Killoran, A. and Seal, H. (1996) *A Framework for Promoting the Health of Older People: a Discussion Document*. London: Centre for Policy on Ageing/Health Education Authority.

Davidson, K. (1996) '"Women grieve, men replace" – myth or reality? Gender differences in the meanings of widowhood', paper presented at the Annual Conference of the British Society of Gerontology, September.

Davies, A. (1990) 'Prevention in the ageing'. In Kane, R., Grimley Evans, J. and Macfadyen, D. (eds). *Improving the Health of Older People: a World View*. Oxford: Oxford University Press.

Deem, R. (1982) 'Women, leisure and inequality', *Leisure Studies*, **1**: 29–46.

Department of Health (1992) *The Health of the Nation: a Strategy for Health in England*, Cm 1986. London: HMSO.

Department of Health (1994) *Report of the Advisory Group on Osteoporosis*. London: DoH.

Department of Health (1996) *Health Related Behaviour: an Epidemiological Overview*. London: HMSO.

Department of Health and Social Security (1980) *Inequalities in Health: Report of a Research Working Group* [the Black Report] London: DHSS.

Department of Health and Social Security (1989) *Mental Illness Statistics, England 1986*. London: HMSO.

Department of Health/Ministry of Agriculture, Fisheries and Food (1997) *National Diet and Nutritional Survey of British Adults aged 65 + years*. Report. London: HMSO.

Donaldson, L. (1986) 'Health and social status of elderly Asians: a community survey', *British Medical Journal*, **293**: 1079–82.

Dooghe, G. (1992) 'Informal caregivers of elderly people: a European overview', *Ageing and Society*, **12**: 369–80.

Downie, R., Fyfe, C. and Tannahill, A. (1992) *Health Promotion: Models and Values*. Oxford: OUP.

Dunne, F. and Schipperheijn, J. (1989) 'Alcohol and the elderly: need for greater awareness', *British Medical Journal*, **298**: 1660–1.

Ebrahim, S., Patel, N., Coats, M., Grieg, C., Gilley, J., Bangham, C. and Stacey, S. (1991) 'Prevalence and severity of morbidity among Gujerati Asian elders: a controlled comparison', *Family Practice*, **8**(1): 57–62.

Edwards, K. and Larson, E. (1992) 'Benefits of exercise for older people', *Clinical Geriatric Medicine*, **8**: 35–52.

Emery, C. and Gatz, M. (1990) 'Psychological and cognitive effects of an exercise programme for community-residing older adults', *Gerontologist*, **30**(2): 184–8.

Emery, C., Hauck, E. R. and Blumenthal, J. A. (1992) 'Exercise adherence or maintenance among older adults: a one year follow up study', *Psychology and Aging*, **7**: 466–70.

Erikson, E., Erikson, J. and Kivnick, H. (1986) *Vital Involvement in Old Age*. New York: Norton.

Fairhurst, E. (1990) 'Doing ethnography in a geriatric unit'. In Peace, S. (ed.), *Researching Social Gerontology: Concepts, Methods and Issues*. London: Sage, chapter 7.

Fennell, G., Phillipson, C. and Evers, H. (1988) *The Sociology of Old Age*. Milton Keynes: Open University Press.

Fenton, S. (1985) *Race, Health and Welfare*. Bristol: University of Bristol.

Ferraro, K. (1985) 'The effect of widowhood on the health status of older persons', *International Journal of Aging and Human Development*, **21**(1): 9–25.

Fielding, N. (1993) 'Qualitative interviewing'. In Gilbert, N. (ed.) *Researching Social Life*. London: Sage, chapter 8.

Fisk, M. and Abbott, S. (1997) *Maintaining independence and involvement: older people speaking*. St Albans: The Abbeyfield Society.

Fox, J. (ed.) (1989) *Health Inequalities in European Countries*. Aldershot: Gower.

Fox, J., Goldblatt, P. and Jones, D. (1983) 'Social class mortality differentials: artefact, selection or life circumstances', *Journal of Epidemiology and Community Health*, **39** (1): 1–18.

Freeman, E. (1994) 'Senior peer counselling: serving a varied and growing population', *Dimensions*, **1**: 2–4.

French, S. (1990) 'Ageism', *Physiotherapy*, **76**(3): 178–82.

Fries, J. (1980) 'Ageing, natural death and the compression of morbidity', *New England Journal of Medicine*, **303**(3): 130–5.

Fries, J. (1989) 'Reduction of the national morbidity'. In Lewis, S. (ed.), *Aging and Health: Linking Research and Public Policy*. Michigan: Lewis, pp. 3–22.

Gibson, (1990) 'Falls in later life.' in Kane, R., Grimley Evans, J. and Macfadyen, D. (eds), *Improving the Health of Older People: a World View*. Oxford: Oxford University Press.

Giddens, A. (1994) *Modernity and Self Identity: Self and Society in the Late Modern Age*. Cambridge: Polity Press.

Ginn, J. and Arber, S. (1995) 'Exploring mid-life women's employment', *Sociology*, **29**(1): 73–94.

Glendenning, F. (1990) 'The health needs of black and ethnic minority elders', *Generations*, **14**: 7–11.

Goddard, E. and Savage, D. (1994) *People aged 65 and over*. OPCS Series GHS No. 22. Supplement A. London: HMSO.

Goldblatt, P. (ed.) (1990) *Longitudinal Study: Mortality and Social Organisation 1971–1981*. OPCS Series LS No. 6. London: HMSO.

Goldman, R. (1994) 'The Survey of Retirement and Retirement Plans: five years on'. *DSS Social Security Yearbook 1993/4*. London: HMSO.

Goldman, N., Korenman, S. and Weinstein, R. (1995) 'Marital status among the elderly', *Social Science and Medicine*, **40**(12): 1717–30.

Gray, M. (ed.) (1985). *Prevention of Disease in the Elderly*. Edinburgh: Churchill Livingstone.

Gray, M. (1986) 'Don't put it down to old age', *Self Health*, **10**: 7–8.

Green, N. M. and Bridgham, J. (1991) 'The older adult alcoholic client'. In Young, R. and Olson, E. (eds), *Health, Illness and Disability in Later Life*. London: Sage, chapter 5.

Gruenberg, E. (1977) 'Failures of success', *Milbank Memorial Quarterly/Health and Society*, **55**: 3–24.

Hakim, C. (1982) *Secondary Analysis in Social Research*. London: Allen & Unwin.

Hall, R. and Channing, D. (1990) 'Age, pattern of consultation and functional disability in elderly patients in one general practice', *British Medical Journal*, **301**(2): 424–7.

Haskell, W. (1997) 'Personal health benefits of exercise for older people'. Research into Ageing's 21st anniversary lecture, presented at the Active for Later Life Conference, Birmingham.

Health Education Authority (1995) *A Survey of the UK Population*, Part 1. London: HEA.

Health Education Authority (1996) *Health and Lifestyles: National Surveys Guide*, CD-Rom. London: HEA.

Henwood, M. (1990) 'No sense of urgency: age discrimination in health care'. In McEwen, E. (ed.) *Age: the Unrecognised Discrimination*. London: Age Concern England.

Hess, J. (1991) 'Health promotion and risk reduction in later life'. In Young and Olson, chapter 2.

Hickey, T. and Stilwell, D. (1991) 'Health promotion for older people: All is not well', *Gerontologist*, **31**(6): 822–9.

Higgs, P. and Victor, C. (1993) 'Institutional care and the life course'. In Arber, S. and Evandrou, M. (eds). *Ageing, Independence and the Life Course*. London: Jessica Kingsley.

Hill, S. (1990) *More than Rice and Peas: Guidelines to Improve Food Provision for Black and Ethnic Minorities in Britain*. London: The Food Commission.

Hopkins, D., Murrah, B., Hoeger, W. and Rhodes, R. (1990) 'Effect of low-impact aerobic dance on the functional fitness of elderly women', *Gerontologist*, **30**(2): 189–92.

Hounslow Leisure Services (1997) *A Matter of Lifestyle: a Study of Asian Communities*. Hounslow: Leisure Services.

Hunter, S. (ed.) (1997) *Dementia: Challenges and New Directions*. London: Jessica Kingsley.

Huppert, F. and Whittington, J. (1993a) 'Longitudinal changes in mental state and personality measures'. In Cox, Huppert and Whichelow, chapter 8.

Huppert, F. and Whittington, J. (1993b) 'Changes in cognitive function in a population sample'. In Cox, Huppert and Whichelow, chapter 9.

Idler, E. and Kasl, S. (1992) 'Religion, disability, depression and the timing of death', *American Journal of Sociology*, **97**(4): 1052–79.

Illsley, R. and Svensson, P. G. (eds) (1990) 'Health inequalities in Europe', *Social Science and Medicine*, Special issue: **31**(3): 225–351.

Isdale, D. (1993) 'Arthritis', *Reviews in Clinical Gerontology*, **3**: 259–80.

Jacobson, B., Smith, A. and Whitehead, M. (eds)(1991) *The Nation's Health: a Strategy for the 1990s*, 2nd edition. London: King Edward's Hospital Fund for London.

Jagger, C., Clarke, M. and Cook, A. (1989) 'Mental and physical health of elderly people: five year follow up of a total population', *Age and Ageing*, **18**(2): 77–82.

Jerrome, D. (1981) 'The significance of friendship for women in later life', *Ageing and Society*, **1**(2): 175–98.

Jerrome, D. (1990) 'Frailty and friendship', *Journal of Cross-cultural Gerontology*, **5**(1): 51–64.

Jowell, R., Witherspoon, S. and Brook, L. (eds) (1990) *British Social Attitudes Survey: 7th Report*. Aldershot: Gower.

Kane, R. L., Grimley Evans, J. and Macfadyen, D. (eds) (1990) *Improving the Health of Older People: a World View*. Oxford: Oxford University Press.

Karp, D. (1988) 'A decade of reminders', *Gerontologist*, **28**(6): 727–38.

Keith, P. (1987) 'Postponement of health care by unmarried older women', *Women and Health*, **12**(1): 47–60.

Kellett, J. (1989) 'The reality of sexual behaviour in old age: There's a lot of it about', *Geriatric Medicine*, **19**(10): 17–18.

King, M. and Tinetti, M. (1995) 'Falls in community-dwelling older persons', *Journal of the American Geriatric Association*, **43**: 1146–54.

King's Fund Institute. (1994) *Analysis of OPCS Omnibus Survey*. London: King's Fund Institute.

Kirkman, M. (1989) 'Nutrition in the elderly', *Physician*, **8**(10): 701–2 and 704.

Koenig, H. (1991) 'Religion and prevention of illness in later life', *Prevention in Human Services*, **10**(1): 69–89.

Koenig, H. (1993) 'Religion and aging', *Reviews in Clinical Gerontology*, **3**(2): 195–203.

Kohli, M., Rein, M., Guillemard, A. M. and van Gunsteren, H. (eds) (1991) *Time for Retirement: Comparative Studies of Early Exit from the Labour Force*. Cambridge: Cambridge University Press.

Kramer, M. (1980) 'The rising pandemic of mental disorders and associated chronic diseases and disabilities', *Acta Psychiatrica Scandinavica*, **285**: 382–97.

Krueger, R. (1994) *Focus Groups: a Practical Guide for Applied Research*. London: Sage.

Laczko, F. and Phillipson, C. (1991) *Changing Work and Retirement: Social Policy and the Older Worker*. Milton Keynes: Open University Press.

Langlie, J. (1977) 'Social networks, health beliefs and preventive health behaviour', *Journal of Health and Social Behaviour*, **18**: 244–60.

Laslett, P. (1989) *A Fresh Map of Life: the Emergence of the Third Age*. London: Weidenfeld & Nicolson.

Levi, L. and Cox, D. (1994) 'Changing the social environment to promote health'. In Abeles, R., Gift, H. and Ory, M. (eds), *Aging and Quality of Life*. New York: Springer, pp. 336–49.

Lindley, C. M., Tully, M. P., Paramsothy, V. and Tallis, R. C.(1992) 'Inappropriate medication is a major cause of adverse drug reactions in elderly patients', *Age and Ageing*, **23**: 294–300.

Lofland, J. (1971) *Analysing Social Settings*. Belmont, Calif.: Wadsworth.

London Research Centre (1997) *The Capital Divided: Mapping Poverty and Social Exclusion in London*. London: LRC.

Lopata, H. (1973) *Widowhood in an American City*. Cambridge, Mass.: Schenkman.

Lowenthal, M. and Haven, C. (1968) 'Interaction and adaptation: intimacy as a critical variable', *American Sociological Review*, **33**(1): 20–30.

Lynn, P. and Lievesley, D. (1991) *Drawing General Population Samples in Great Britain*. London: Social and Community Planning Research.

McCormick, A. and Rosenbaum, M. (1990) *Morbidity Statistics from General Practice, Third National Study: Socioeconomic Analysis*. Series MB5, No. 2. London: HMSO.

Macdonald, A. (1986) 'Do general practitioners "miss" depression in elderly patients?', *British Medical Journal*, **292**: 1365–7.

McIsaac, S. (1995) ' "Interviewing" confused older people', *Generations Review*, **5**(4): 4–5.

McManus, L. (1985) *Hypothermia: the Facts*. Mitcham: Age Concern England.

McMurdo, M. and Johnstone, R. (1995) 'A randomised controlled trial of a home exercise programme for elderly people with poor mobility', *Age and Ageing*, **24**: 425–8.

Manton, K. G. (1988) 'A longitudinal study of functional change and mortality in the US', *Journal of Gerontology*, **43**(5): 153–61.

Manton, K. G., Stallard, E. and Corder, L. (1995) 'Changes in morbidity and chronic disability in the U.S. elderly population: evidence from the 1982, 1984 and 1989 National Long Term Care Survey', *Journal of Gerontology*, **50B**, S104–S204.

Markides, K. (ed.) (1989) *Aging and Health: Perspectives on Gender, Race, Ethnicity and Class*. Newbury Park, Calif.: Sage.

Marmot, M., Adelstein, A. and Bulusi, L. (1984) *Immigrant Mortality in England and Wales: 1970–1978*, OPCS Studies on Population and Medical Subjects No. 47. London: HMSO.

Martin Matthews, A. and Campbell, L. (1995) 'Gender roles, employment and informal care'. In Arber, S. and Ginn, J. (eds), *Connecting Gender and Ageing*. Buckingham: Open University Press, chapter 10.

Martin, J., Meltzer, H. and Elliot, D. (1988) *OPCS Surveys of Disability in Great Britain: Report 1 – The Prevalence of Disability Among Adults*. London: HMSO.

Mays, N. (1994) ' "Race" and health in contemporary Britain (review)', *British Medical Journal*, **309**: 67.

Medical Research Council (1994) *The Health of the UK's Elderly People*. London: MRC.

Miller, M. (1986) 'Factors promoting wellness in the aged person: an ethnographic study', *Advanced Nursing Science*, **13**(4): 38–51.

Miller, M. (1991) 'Drug use and misuse among the elderly'. In Young, R. and Olson, E. (eds) *Health, Illness and Disability in Later Life: Practice Issues and Interventions*. London: Sage, chapter 3.

Morgan, D. (1988) *Focus Groups as Qualitative Research*. London: Sage.

Morgan, D. (1993) *Successful Focus Groups: Advancing the State of the Art*. London: Sage.

Morris, M. (1986) 'Music and movement for the elderly', *Nursing Times*, **83**(8): 44–5.

Morton, J. (ed.) (1993) *Recent Research on Services for Black and Minority Ethnic Elderly People*, Report of proceedings of the Ageing Update Conference, London, July 1992. London: Age Concern Institute of Gerontology.

Muir Gray, J. (ed.) (1985) *Prevention of Disease in the Elderly*. Edinburgh: Churchill Livingstone.

Murphy, E. (1982) 'Social origins of depression in old age', *British Journal of Psychiatry*, **141**: 135–42.

Nathanson, C. A. (1975) 'Illness and the feminine role: a theoretical review', *Social Science and Medicine*, **9**: 57–62.

Nathanson, C. A. (1977) 'Sex, illness and medical care: a review of the data, theory and method', *Social Science and Medicine*, **11**: 13–25.

Nettleton, S. (1996) 'Women and the new paradigm of health and medicine', *Critical Social Policy*, **16**(3): 33–53.

Norman, A. (1985) *Triple Jeopardy: Growing Old in a Second Homeland*. London: Centre for Policy on Ageing.

ONS (1997a) *Social Trends 27*. London: Stationery Office.

ONS (1997b) *Living in Britain: Results from the 1995 General Household Survey*. London: Stationery Office.

OPCS (1986) 'Hypothermia deaths', *Population Trends 44*: 2–4.

OPCS (1990) *Population Trends 61*. London: HMSO.

OPCS (1993) *Communal Establishments, 1991 Census*. London: HMSO.

OPCS (1994) *Census 1991 Communal Establishments, Great Britain*. London: HMSO.

OPCS (1996) *Population Trends 86*. London: HMSO.

Orrell, M. and Sahakin, B. (1995) 'Education and dementia: Research evidence supports the concept of "use it or lose it"', *British Medical Journal*, **310**: 951–2.

Peace, S. (ed.) (1990) *Researching Social Gerontology: Concepts, Methods and Issues*. London: Sage.

Perrson, O. and Skoog, I. (1996) 'Prospective population study of psychosocial risk factors for late onset dementia', *International Journal of Geriatric Psychology*, **11**: 15–22.

Procter, M. (1993) 'Measuring attitudes'. In Gilbert, N. *Researching Social Life*. London: Sage, pp. 116–34.

Qureshi, H. (1990) 'Social support'. In Peace, S. (ed.), *Researching Social Gerontology: Concepts, Methods and Issues*. London: Sage, pp. 32–45.

Raleigh, S. (1992) *Health Care for Ethnic Minority Older People*, Fact Sheet No. 3. Guildford: Institute of Public Health/King's Fund Centre.

Ripich, D. and Terrell, B. (1988) 'Patterns of discourse cohesion and coherence in Alzheimer's Disease', *Journal of Speech and Hearing Disorders*, **53**(1): 8–15.

Roberts, A. (1989) 'Sexuality in later life', *Nursing Times*, **85**(24): 65–8.

Roberts, S. and Boardman, B. (1989) 'Beating the cold: the role of social services', *Social Work Today*, **20**(19): 20–1.

Rogers, R., Meyer, J. and Mortel, K. (1990) 'After reaching retirement age physical activity sustains cerebral perfusion and cognition', *Journal of the American Geriatrics Society*, **38**(2): 123–8.

Rose, G. (1992) *The Strategy of Preventive Medicine*. Oxford: Oxford University Press.

Royal College of Physicians (1992) *Preventive Medicine: a Report of a Working Party of the RCP*. London: RCP.

Sidell, M. (1991) *Gender Differences in the Health of Older People*, Research Report, Department of Health and Social Welfare. Milton Keynes: Open University.

Sidell, M. (1995) *Health in Old Age: Myth, Mystery and Management*. Buckingham: Open University Press.

Silverman, P. (1986) *Widow-to-widow*. New York: Springer.

Smaje, C. (1995) *Health, 'Race' and Ethnicity: Making Sense of the Evidence*. London: King's Fund Institute.

Stanfield, J. (1993), 'Methodological reflections: an introduction'. In Stanfield, J. and Dennis, R. (eds) *Race and Ethnicity in Research Methods*. London: Sage, pp. 3–15.

Svanborg, A. (1988) 'The health of the elderly population: results from longitudinal studies with age cohort comparisons'. In Evered, D. and Whelan, J. (eds), *Research and the Ageing Population*. London: Wiley.

Swain, V. (1993a) 'Changing views on health and ill-health'. In Cox, Huppert and Whichelow, chapter 16.

Swain, V. (1993b) 'Social relationships and health'. In Cox, Huppert and Whichelow, chapter 15.

Tarpey, M. (1990) 'Service provision to elderly people from black and ethnic minority groups', *Generations*, **14**: 11–16.

Taylor, R. (1988) 'The elderly as members of society: an examination of social differences in an elderly population'. In Wells, N. and Freer, C. (eds), *The Ageing Population – Burden or Challenge?* Basingstoke: Macmillan, pp. 105–29

Taylor, Marcia Freed (1992) *British Household Panel Survey User Manual*, volume A: Introduction, technical report and appendices. Colchester: University of Essex.

Thoits, P. (1982) 'Conceptual methodological and theoretical problems in studying social support as a buffer against life stress', *Journal of Health and Social Behaviour*, **23**: 145.

Thornton, P. and Tozer, R. (1994) *Involving Older People in Planning and Evaluating Community Care: a Review of Initiatives*. York: Social Policy Research Unit.

Tinetti, M., Baker, D., Mcavay, G., Claus, E., Garrett, P., Gottshalk, M., Koch, M., Trainor, K. and Horwitz, R. (1994) 'A multifactorial intervention to reduce the risk of falling among elderly people living in the community', *New England Journal of Medicine*, **331**: 821–7.

Tones, B. (1981) 'Affective education and health'. In Crowley, J., David, K. and Williams, T. (eds), *Health Education in Schools*. London: Harper & Row.

Townsend, P., Davidson, N. and Whitehead, M. (1988) *Inequalities in Health and the Health Divide*. Harmondsworth: Penguin.

Townsend, P., Phillimore, P. and Beattie, A. (1988) *Health and Deprivation: Inequality and the North*. London: Croom Helm.

Tudor-Hart, J. (1971) 'The inverse care law', *Lancet*, **1**(696): 405–12.

van de Water, H. (1997) 'Healthy active life expectancy and the problem of substitute morbidity', paper presented to meeting, 'Ageing: Science, Medicine and Society', 7–8 May at The Royal Society, London.

Verbrugge, L. (1984a) 'A health profile of older women with comparisons to older men', *Research on Aging*, **6**: 291–322.

Verbrugge, L. (1984b) 'Longer life but worsening health? Trends in health and mortality of middle aged and older persons', *Milbank Memorial Fund Quarterly/Health and Society*, **62**(3): 475–519.

Verbrugge, L. (1989) 'Gender, aging and health' In Markides, K (ed.), *Aging and Health: Perspectives on Gender, Race, Ethnicity and Class.* Newbury Park, Calif.: Sage, pp. 23–78.

Vetter, N. (1989) 'Why persuading the elderly to give up smoking is worthwhile', *Pulse*, January.

Victor, C. (1991) 'Continuity or change: inequalities in health in later life', *Ageing and Society*, **11**(1): 23–39.

Victor, C. (in press) *Promoting the Health of Older People*, Report of an HEA Expert Group. London: HEA.

Victor, C. and Evandrou, M. (1987) 'Does social class matter in later life?' In Di Gregorio, S. (ed.), *Social Gerontology: New Directions.* London: Croom Helm, pp. 252–67

Wagner, E., Lacroix, A., Grothaus, L., Leveille, S., Hecht, J., Artz, K., Odle, K. and Buchner, D. (1994) 'Preventing disability and falls in older adults: a population based randomised trial', *American Journal of Public Health*, **84**: 1800–6.

Waldron, I. (1976) 'Why do women live longer than men?' *Social Science and Medicine*, **10**: 349–62.

Wallace, R. (1994) 'Assessing the health of individuals and populations in surveys of the elderly: some concepts and approaches', *Gerontologist*, **14**(4): 449–53.

Welch, J. (1990) 'AIDS in the elderly: What aims for HIV testing?', *Geriatric Medicine*, **20**(2): 9.

Wenger, C. (1989) 'Support networks in old age: constructing a typology'. In Jefferys, M. (ed.), *Growing Old in the Twentieth Century.* London: Routledge.

Whichelow, M. (1993a) 'Changes in dietary habits'. In Cox, Huppert and Whichelow, chapter 11.

Whichelow, M. (1993b) 'Trends in alcohol consumption'. In Cox, Huppert and Whichelow, chapter 13.

Whichelow, M. and Cox, B. (1993) 'Alterations in smoking patterns'. In Cox, Huppert and Whichelow, chapter 12.

White, A., Nicolaas, G., Foster, K., Browne, F. and Carey, S. (1993) *Health Survey for England 1991.* Social Survey Division of OPCS. London: HMSO.

Whitehead, M. (1987) *The Health Divide: Inequalities in Health in the 1980s.* London: Health Education Council.

Whittington, J. and Huppert, F. (1993) 'The impact of life events on wellbeing'. In Cox, Huppert and Whichelow, chapter 10.

Windle, R. and Mouncey, P. (1997) 'Non-response and public perception of market research', Market Research Society Conference, 1997 Conference Papers.

Wise, G. (1986) 'Overcoming loneliness', *Nursing Times*, **82**(22): 37–42.

World Health Organisation (1983) 'The elderly in eleven countries: a sociomedical survey', *Public Health in Europe No. 21*. Copenhagen: WHO Regional Office for Europe.

World Health Organisation (1985) *Targets for Health for All, 2000*. Copenhagen: WHO.

World Health Organisation (1991) *Targets for Health for All, 2000*, Copenhagen: WHO.

World Health Organisation (1992a) *Approaches to Stress Management in the Community Setting*. Report on a WHO consultation. Copenhagen: WHO Regional Office for Europe.

World Health Organisation (1992b) *Health Aspects Related to Indoor Air Quality*. Report on a WHO Working Group. Copenhagen: WHO.

World Health Organisation (1993) *Health for All Targets: the Health Policy for Europe*. Copenhagen: WHO Regional Office for Europe.

World Health Organisation (1995) *Epidemiology and Prevention of Cardiovascular Disease in Older People*. Geneva: WHO.

Wright, F. (1997) *Ageing Well: the Pros and Cons of Health Volunteers*. London: Age Concern Institute of Gerontology/Department of Health.

Young, R. and Olson, E. (1991) *Health, Illness and Disability in Later Life: Practice Issues and Interventions*. London: Sage.